# Morphine and Metastasis

Marie-Odile Parat
Editor

# Morphine and Metastasis

Springer

*Editor*
Marie-Odile Parat
School of Pharmacy
University of Queensland
Woolloongabba
Australia

ISBN 978-94-007-5677-9 ISBN 978-94-007-5678-6 (eBook)
DOI 10.1007/978-94-007-5678-6
Springer Dordrecht Heidelberg New York London

Library of Congress Control Number: 2012951126



Printed on acid-free paper

Springer is part of Springer Science+Business Media (www.springer.com)

# Contents

# Chapter 1
# Morphine and Metastasis: From Bench to Bedside

**Marie-Odile Parat**

**Abstract** The possibility that morphine and other opioids may modulate tumour growth and metastasis has been researched for many years. The recent past has seen multiple clinical studies attempting to document whether limiting the perioperative use of morphine is beneficial for cancer surgery patients. Furthermore, a lot of exciting new data has been generated in vitro, but also in preclinical and clinical studies, that indirectly shed light on the effect of opioids on cancer. Future directions in the field may include the role of endogenous morphine in tumour biology, the recent discovery that genetic polymorphisms of the mu opioid receptor are associated with cancer survival, the role of microRNAs in opioid receptor regulation and signalling, and the potential usefulness of peripheral opioid antagonists.

**Keywords** Cancer • Endogenous morphine • Immunosuppression • Methylnaltrexone • MicroRNA • Morphine glucuronides • Opioid antagonists • Opioid receptor • Pain management • Polymorphism • Surgery • Tolerance • Tumor microenvironment • Withdrawal

## Abbreviations

| | |
|---|---|
| MOR | μ opioid receptor |
| bFGF | basic fibroblast growth factor |
| CABG | coronary artery bypass grafting |
| EGFR | epidermal growth factor receptor |
| MiRNAs | micro ribonucleic acids |

M.-O. Parat (✉)
School of Pharmacy, Pharmacy Australia Centre of Excellence, University of Queensland, 20 Cornwall Street, Woolloongabba, QLD 4102, Australia

Outcomes Research Consortium, Cleveland, OH, USA
e-mail: m.parat@uq.edu.au

M.-O. Parat (ed.), *Morphine and Metastasis*, DOI 10.1007/978-94-007-5678-6_1, 

| | |
|---|---|
| M3G | morphine-3-glucuronide |
| M6G | morphine-6-glucuronide |
| MD2 | myeloid differentiation protein-2 |
| NO | nitric oxide |
| NOS | nitric oxide synthase |
| NOP | nociceptin receptor |
| PDGFRβ | platelet-derived growth factor receptor β |
| RT-PCR | reverse transcriptase polymerase chain reaction |
| TLR4 | toll-like receptor 4 |
| UTR | untranslated region |
| VEGFR | vascular endothelial growth factor receptor |
| DOR | δ opioid receptor |
| KOR | κ opioid receptor |

## 1.1 Introduction

A vast research effort is currently being carried out by a variety of scientists and clinicians to determine whether opioids, and in particular morphine, influence the growth and metastasis of tumours with obvious clinical implications: morphine is administered to cancer patients to alleviate their pain, and most often as part of the perioperative pain management of solid tumour surgical ablation.

Research shows a variety of effects for morphine and other opioids depending on the complexity of the system studied: cell, tumour and its micro-environment, entire body. At the cellular level, the various receptors and signalling pathways involved, the dose responses, the chronicity of exposure and the opioids tested already engender some discrepancies in the reported effect of opioids on cancer cells, as well as other cell types important in tumour growth such as endothelial cells or immune cells (Afsharimani et al. 2011a). Animal studies have tested the impact of morphine in rodents implanted with tumour cells in the absence of surgical stress, or concomitant with laparotomy, with there again contradicting results (Afsharimani et al. 2011b). It is clear that in the context of pain, the potential growth and metastasis-promoting effects of morphine are offset by its pain-killing effects – pain being a much worse tumour-promoting factor (Page et al. 1993, 1998, 2001; Sasamura et al. 2002). Extrapolation of animal studies to the clinical context is delicate given the difference in morphine metabolism between mice and humans (Hoskin et al. 1989; Kuo et al. 1991). Lastly, clinical studies testing the effect of morphine on tumour growth or metastasis in a non-surgical context are inexistent but recently, a number of retrospective studies and one prospective trial have tested the role of perioperative anaesthesia and pain management on cancer recurrence or metastasis in cancer surgery patients (reviewed in Shilling and Tiouririne (2013), Popping et al. (2013), Shanahan et al. (2013)) – perioperative pain management includes multiple variable factors, one of which is the use of opioid analgesics. Ultimately, research on the effect of opioid on cancer growth, metastasis, and post-surgical recurrence will serve to establish guidelines regarding the use of opioids in cancer patients.

## 1.2 Morphine and Tumour Growth and Metastasis at the Cell Level

In addition to their ability to control pain via centrally mediated pathways, opioids can act peripherally, on cells that can directly influence tumour growth or metastasis especially cancer cells, endothelial cells, and immune cells. While mostly attributed to opioid actions on the μ, κ, δ opioid classical receptors (MOR, KOR, DOR, respectively), some of the effects of opioids on tumour or cancer-associated cells are hypothesized to be non opioid receptor-mediated when they are experimentally not reversed – or only partially – by pharmacological antagonists or by molecular receptor ablation (Afsharimani et al. 2011a). In some cases, direct actions of opioids on non-opioid receptors have been identified. Naloxone competes with 17β-estradiol for binding to the estrogen receptor and acts as an antagonist of estrogen receptor activity, with obvious therapeutic implications in estrogen-dependent tumours (Farooqui et al. 2006; Johnson et al. 2013). In other cases, opioids can transactivate, via action through opioid receptors, growth factor receptors relevant to cancer growth: morphine-induced phosphorylation of the epidermal growth factor receptor (EGFR) occurs via opioid receptors and the coactivation of EGFR by opioid receptors can be antagonized by naloxone (Fujioka et al. 2011). Opioid receptors also transactivate platelet-derived growth factor receptor β (PDGFRβ) (Chen et al. 2006; Wang et al. 2012d) and vascular endothelial growth factor receptors (VEGFR) (Singleton et al. 2006; Chen et al. 2006) and the downstream signalling and functional consequences of growth factor receptor transactivation can be inhibited by opioid receptor antagonism (Singleton et al. 2006).

Other receptors may be of relevance to the effect of opioids on tumour growth and metastasis. Morphine has been shown to stimulate nitric oxide (NO) release by constitutive nitric oxide synthase (NOS) in macrophages and endothelial cells – important players of the tumour microenvironment – and this is proposed to occur via a novel alternatively spliced variant of the MOR named μ3 (Stefano et al. 1995; Cadet et al. 2004). The expression of this receptor has been evidenced in cancer tissue via binding and reverse transcriptase polymerase chain reaction (RT-PCR) assays (Fimiani et al. 1999). Moreover, morphine is proposed to activate inflammation via activation of the Toll-like receptor 4 (TLR4) through binding of the TLR4-associated protein myeloid differentiation protein-2 (MD2) on central nervous system endothelial and microglial cells (Wang et al. 2012c). Actions of opioids on TRL4 of tumour cells (Hassan et al. 2006; Molteni et al. 2006; Tang et al. 2010) or surrounding endothelial cells or macrophages can be hypothesized to similarly modulate the tumour microenvironment. Therefore, in addition to affecting cellular responses such as proliferation, apoptosis, migration and invasion, opioids have the potential to modulate angiogenesis (Gupta 2013), inflammation, vascular integrity (Lennon and Singleton 2013), the immune response (Koodie and Roy 2013), and thus determine the tumour microenvironment.

Little is known about opioids in the tumour microenvironment – Opioids may be able to modulate the cross talk between cancer and non-cancer cells within the tumour (Fuggetta et al. 2005). The MOR expression is increased in some tumour cell lines and in tumour samples (Mathew et al. 2011). Morphine has been shown to down-regulate basic fibroblast growth factor (bFGF) production in human monocyte-derived macrophages (Dave and Khalili 2010). Moreover, the endogenous opioid production by immune cells, providing analgesia at sites of inflammation (Cabot et al. 1997), is likely to be relevant to immune cells in the tumour microenvironment but this has not been explored in a cancer-specific setting.

## 1.3 At the Animal Level

Many studies have shown discrepant results when testing the effect of opioids on rodent tumour models, ranging from a net tumour-promoting effect (Ishikawa et al. 1993; Gupta et al. 2002) to inhibition of tumour growth (Yeager and Colacchio 1991; Sasamura et al. 2002; Koodie et al. 2010). Mouse studies need to be examined keeping in mind that many genetic variations in the μ-opioid receptor gene between wild-derived mouse strains are associated with differences in opioid sensitivity (Shigeta et al. 2008). Similarly, genetic variation between mouse strains can be hypothesized to explain – at least in part – the variations in the effect of opioids on tumour growth or angiogenesis between different research groups and published studies. Additional variability between studies can be attributed to differences in experimental conditions as reviewed elsewhere (Afsharimani et al. 2011a). When rodents are subjected to pain or surgical stress in addition to being inoculated with tumour cells, morphine is protective against tumour growth and/or metastasis (Page et al. 1993, 1994, 1998; Bar-Yosef et al. 2001; Sasamura et al. 2002). Therefore, providing the best possible pain relief to cancer patients may influence disease outcome.

## 1.4 At the Bedside

One of the problems in extending findings from preclinical studies to humans is the fact that there are wide species differences in morphine glucuronidation and in particular, between humans and rodents: humans metabolise morphine into morphine-6-glucuronide (M6G) which is a more potent analgesic than morphine, and is found in the circulation in concentrations exceeding those of morphine itself after parenteral or oral administration (Osborne et al. 1988, 1990), and morphine-3-glucuronide

(M3G) which loses analgesic effect (Shimomura et al. 1971). In contrast, mice and rats produce mostly M3G. This was determined through urinary excretion of metabolites, and ratios of the metabolising enzyme uridine diphosphate-glucuronyltransferase activities towards the −3 and −6 hydroxyl groups of morphine in liver microsomes (Kuo et al. 1991), although production of M6G in rat brain tissue seems higher (Nagano et al. 2000). As a consequence of this difference in metabolism, rodents require doses in mg/kg that are much higher than humans and "clinically relevant" doses of morphine employed in rodents should take into account the concentrations and pharmacokinetics of active morphine metabolites. Furthermore, the contribution of morphine and its metabolites to the modulation of tumour growth and metastasis has not often been dissected out. In a study documenting the pro-angiogenic effect of opioids in vitro, activation of endothelial cell migration was demonstrated for morphine and M6G but not M3G (Singleton et al. 2006). It has been suggested that morphine metabolites M6G and M3G modulate immune responses in cancer patients, although the study did not elucidate whether the metabolites acted on humoral and cellular immunity or whether they were just a reflection of morphine intake (Hashiguchi et al. 2005). In contrast, in rats administered with exogenous M6G, suppression of immune function was demonstrated and suggested to be centrally mediated (Carrigan and Lysle 2001).

A second issue in determining from clinical studies whether opioids actually modulate tumour growth, metastasis or recurrence in patients undergoing tumour resection is the complexity of the perioperative factors, difficult to control for. In prospective or retrospective studies comparing regional analgesia to opioid-based analgesia, opioid intake is not the only factor that differs between groups (Exadaktylos et al. 2006; Biki et al. 2008; Sessler et al. 2008; Tsui et al. 2010; Wuethrich et al. 2010; Myles et al. 2011, De Oliveira et al. 2011, Forget et al. 2011, Cummings et al. 2012, Day et al. 2012). Indirect approaches may therefore be necessary to shed light on the role of opioids in tumour growth and metastasis, for example by studying the association between genetic polymorphisms influencing opioid function and cancer survival (Bortsov et al. 2012, 2013).

## 1.5 Additional Factors That Engender Variability

Additional factors that may be responsible for variability in published data about the effect of opioid on tumour growth and metastasis include the acute versus chronic exposure to opioids. In cell culture studies, morphine is mostly applied for a maximum of a few days before measurement of the endpoint. In animals, osmotic pumps, morphine-releasing pellets or repeated subcutaneous or intraperitoneal injections every 12 h have been used over very different periods of time. In the clinical setting, perioperative pain and chronic pain of cancer patients are managed differently. It is known that chronic use of morphine and other opioids produces tolerance and dependence via adaptations in the nervous system and peripheral tissues at multiple levels (compensatory changes in signal transduction leading to alterations in gene transcription, levels of second messengers and neurotransmitters). These adaptive changes have been proposed to be initiated through endocytic trafficking of activated receptors (Martini and Whistler 2007). Research in this area has mostly targeted central nervous system cell types. To which extent the effects of opioids on tumour growth and metastasis can be modulated by chronic versus acute use is largely unknown. Most animal studies assessing the effects of opioid administration on immune function (which is thought to mediate some of the effects of opioids on tumour growth and metastasis) have employed acute or subacute (not sufficient to induce marked dependence or tolerance) administration (Eisenstein et al. 2006). In this context, opioids are mostly immunosuppressive. However, some studies have shown that long term exposure to opioids can lead to tolerance to some (including NK cell activity), but not all, parameters of immune suppression, i.e. some immune parameters that are suppressed during acute exposure to opioids return to normal as the time of exposure increases (Eisenstein et al. 1998). This may translate into a different effect in cancer patients treated with perioperative or chronic morphine. Interestingly, opioid withdrawal in dependent animals or long term opioid users is associated with suppressed immunity (Eisenstein et al. 1998).

## 1.6 Future Directions

### *1.6.1 Endogenous Morphine*

In addition to exogenously administered morphine, the study of morphine in relation to tumour growth and metastasis should take into account the increasingly recognized existence of endogenous morphine, the biological and physio-pathological implications of which are still not fully understood (Stefano et al. 2012). Animal and human cells are now known to be able to produce low concentrations of endogenous, genuine morphine (Poeaknapo et al. 2004; Boettcher et al. 2005). A biological role for endogenous morphine is supported by the existence of μ3 and μ4 opioid receptors, which respond to opiate alkaloids such as morphine but not to the previously recognized endogenous opioid peptides (Stefano et al. 2012). The production of endogenous morphine is not restricted to neuronal cells. Some of the cells tested so far and shown to produce morphine in vitro include immune cells (Zhu et al. 2005; Glattard et al. 2010) and various cancer cell lines (Poeaknapo et al. 2004; Muller et al. 2008).

At this stage a potential role for endogenous morphine in modulating cancer growth and metastasis is entirely speculative and comes from the juxtaposition of (i) knowledge of the existence of endogenous morphine and (ii) data on the effect of exogenous morphine on cancer. Whether cancer cells or non-cancer stroma cells produce and respond to endogenous morphine, with the potential for autocrine or paracrine signalling within the tumour micro-environment is unanswered. Clinical data on circulating levels of endogenous morphine in cancer patients are lacking. In an early study, Munjal et al. determined that normal lung tissue and non-cancerous lung cell lines produced endogenous morphine whereas lung cancer cell lines (both small cell and non-small cell lines) did not, therefore hypothesizing that endogenous morphine could prevent cell proliferation in the context of lung cancer (Munjal et al. 1995).

Of interest to our topic, endogenous morphine production is elicited in humans by surgery and is proposed to be part of the surgical stress response. Plasma morphine concentrations were shown to be significantly elevated from postoperative days 1–5 following coronary artery bypass grafting (CABG) surgery in patients receiving no exogenous morphine (Brix-Christensen et al. 1997). Cardiopulmonary bypass in itself was shown to elicit postoperative morphine production in neonatal pigs, while sham operated animals, undergoing sternotomy without cardiopulmonary bypass, had no detectable endogenous morphine (Brix-Christensen et al. 2000). The involvement of surgical stress in the increased endogenous morphine production was demonstrated by comparing laparoscopic procedures to open laparotomy: in two studies of cholecystectomy and colectomy, respectively, open surgery resulted in significantly higher endogenous morphine concentrations than laparoscopic surgery (Yoshida et al. 2000; Madbouly et al. 2010). It has been proposed, based on the immunosuppressive effects shown for exogenous morphine, that endogenous morphine may be part of the body anti-inflammatory response to the trauma of surgery (Brix-Christensen et al. 1997).

### *1.6.2 Opioid Receptor Polymorphisms*

Over 700 genetic polymorphisms of the mu opioid receptor gene (OPRM1) have been identified in humans, and shown to be associated with opioid sensitivity, substance dependence and susceptibility to other disorders (Kasai and Ikeda 2011). The most abundantly studied OPRM1 SNP, A118G, results for G-allele carriers in a decreased sensitivity to opioid analgesia – and subsequent decrease in pain relief, increase in morphine requirement, and increased opioid consumption, demonstrated both in post-operative pain and cancer pain studies (reviewed in (Kasai and Ikeda 2011). Disorders that have been associated with the A118G polymorphism of the OPRM1 gene include epilepsy and schizophrenia, where the G-allele may be a risk, and diabetes and obesity, where the G-allele may be protective (reviewed in (Kasai and Ikeda 2011). Recently, exciting data has been generated indicating that genetic polymorphisms of the μ opioid receptor and thus presumably variations in opioid signalling may be involved in cancer. Bortsov et al. have studied the association of A118G with breast cancer survival and showed that women with one or more copies of the G-allele had decreased breast cancer-specific mortality (Bortsov et al. 2012, 2013). Opioid intake – which can be hypothesized to be higher in carriers of the G-allele (Klepstad et al. 2004; Chou et al. 2006; Campa et al. 2007; Sia et al. 2008) – was no reported in that study. Studying the same SNP, Wang et al. further demonstrated that carrying the G-allele was associated with a significantly reduced risk for esophageal squamous cell carcinoma (Wang et al. 2012a). Whether these associations are directly linked to the effect of opioid signalling on tumour biology, or influence cancer indirectly via other disorders (such as obesity) or risk factors (such as tobacco dependence) will no doubt be researched in the coming years. Given that prospective trials directly studying whether opioids affect cancer may not be feasible, this field may provide useful, indirect answers about the role of opioids on cancer outcome.

### *1.6.3 Opioid Receptor Antagonists*

Being able to antagonize the potentially harmful peripheral effects of morphine on tumour growth and metastasis while preserving central pain relief which is known to inhibit tumour growth and metastasis has been proposed as a course of action to manage cancer pain while optimizing side effects of opioid agonists. Indeed, peripheral-specific antagonists have been shown to be of benefit regarding unwanted peripheral side effects such as constipation (Yuan et al. 1996) without altering the central analgesia obtained with morphine treatment. It is thus interesting to hypothesize that in models where morphine promotes tumour growth or metastasis, the concomitant administration of a peripheral opioid antagonist will provide protection. In fact, cancer growth and metastasis have been shown to be prevented by MOR antagonism in an animal tumour model independent from morphine administration (Mathew et al. 2011).

### *1.6.4 Exploring the Role of MicroRNAs in Morphine Effect on Cancer*

Micro ribonucleic acids (miRNAs) are small non-coding RNA molecules involved in post transcriptional regulation of gene expression via binding to partially complementary sequences in the 3′ untranslated region (UTR) of target mRNA transcripts, resulting in decreased polypeptide synthesis. Alterations in miRNA expression are known to modulate tumorigenesis, tumour aggressiveness, invasion, metastasis, and tumour sensitivity to treatment (Schoof et al. 2012). Interestingly, morphine and other mu opioid agonists regulate miRNA expression in neuronal (Zheng et al. 2010) and non-neuronal (Dave and Khalili 2010) cells. The morphine-induced increase in miRNA-15b expression in human monocyte-derived macrophages was shown to result in decreased expression of the essential pro-angiogenic growth factor bFGF (Dave and Khalili 2010). Morphine further increased miRNAs of the Let-7 family in the neuronal SH-SY5Y neuronal cell line but also in vivo in a mouse model (He et al. 2010). Let-7 miRNAs are down-regulated in many cancers and have been generally found to be tumour suppressors, inhibiting cell proliferation and survival by affecting a number of oncogenes, cell cycle regulators, cell differentiation and apoptotic pathways mediators, such that let-7 upregulation is proposed to be an effective therapeutic target in cancer (Thornton and Gregory 2012; Boyerinas et al. 2010; Wang et al. 2012b). Whether morphine-induced upregulation of Let-7 may result in altered growth of tumour cells is unexplored at present.

Conversely, expression of the MOR is regulated by miRNAs. An *in silico* search for miRNAs that may interact with the 3'UTR of the MOR mRNA identified the let-7 family of miRNAs as top candidates (He and Wang 2012). Knock-down experiments confirmed that MOR expression is controlled by let-7. Therefore, morphine induces let-7 expression which in turn down-regulates the expression of the MOR. This has been shown to result in opioid tolerance in neuronal cells and in mice (He et al. 2010). Whether a similar mechanism may regulate tumour cell response to opioids is entirely unknown.

## 1.7 Concluding Remarks

Optimal pain management of cancer patients is of the utmost importance, and may influence disease outcome. Current investigations and cross talk between basic science and clinical trials will refine our understanding of the multiple levels of actions of morphine and other opioids on tumour growth and metastasis, and result in improved guidelines for patient care.

**Acknowledgements** We are grateful to Peter J. Cabot for critically reading the manuscript.

## References

Afsharimani B, Cabot PJ, Parat MO (2011a) Morphine and tumor growth and metastasis. Cancer Metastasis Rev 30:225–238

Afsharimani B, Cabot PJ, Parat MO (2011b) Morphine use in cancer surgery. Front Pharmacol 2:46

Bar-Yosef S, Melamed R, Page GG, Shakhar G, Shakhar K, Ben-Eliyahu S (2001) Attenuation of the tumor-promoting effect of surgery by spinal blockade in rats. Anesthesiology 94:1066–1073

Biki B, Mascha E, Moriarty DC, Fitzpatrick JM, Sessler DI, Buggy DJ (2008) Anesthetic technique for radical prostatectomy surgery affects cancer recurrence: a retrospective analysis. Anesthesiology 109:180–187

Boettcher C, Fellermeier M, Boettcher C, Drager B, Zenk MH (2005) How human neuroblastoma cells make morphine. Proc Natl Acad Sci USA 102:8495–8500

Bortsov AV, Millikan RC, Belfer I, Boortz-Marx RL, Arora H, McLean SA (2012) Mu-opioid receptor gene A118G polymorphism predicts survival in patients with breast cancer. Anesthesiology 116:896–902

Bortsov AV, Millikan RC, Belfer I, Boortz-Marx RL, Arora H, McLean SL (2013) Genetic polymorphisms in the μ-opioid receptor gene and breast cancer survival. In: Parat MO (ed) Morphine and metastasis. Springer, Dordrecht

Boyerinas B, Park SM, Hau A, Murmann AE, Peter ME (2010) The role of let-7 in cell differentiation and cancer. Endocr Relat Cancer 17:F19–F36

Brix-Christensen V, Tonnesen E, Sanchez RG, Bilfinger TV, Stefano B (1997) Endogenous morphine levels increase following cardiac surgery as part of the antiinflammatory response? Int J Cardiol 62:191–197

Brix-Christensen V, Goumon Y, Tonnesen E, Chew M, Bilfinger T, Stefano GB (2000) Endogenous morphine is produced in response to cardiopulmonary bypass in neonatal pigs. Acta Anaesthesiol Scand 44:1204–1208

Cabot PJ, Carter L, Gaiddon C, Zhang Q, Schafer M, Loeffler JP, Stein C (1997) Immune cell-derived beta-endorphin: production, release, and control of inflammatory pain in rats. J Clin Invest 100:142–148

Cadet P, Rasmussen M, Zhu W, Tonnesen E, Mantione KJ, Stefano GB (2004) Endogenous morphinergic signaling and tumor growth. Front Biosci 9:3176–3186

Campa D, Gioia A, Tomei A, Poli P, Barale R (2007) Association of ABCB1//MDR1 and OPRM1 Gene Polymorphisms with Morphine Pain Relief. Clin Pharmacol Ther 83:559–566

Carrigan KA, Lysle DT (2001) Morphine-6-beta-glucuronide induces potent immunomodulation. Int Immunopharmacol 1:821–831

Chen C, Farooqui M, Gupta K (2006) Morphine stimulates vascular endothelial growth factor-like signaling in mouse retinal endothelial cells. Curr Neurovasc Res 3:171–180

Chou WY, Wang CH, Liu PH, Liu CC, Tseng CC, Jawan B (2006) Human opioid receptor A118G polymorphism affects intravenous patient-controlled analgesia morphine consumption after total abdominal hysterectomy. Anesthesiology 105:334–337

Cummings KC III, Xu F, Cummings LC, Cooper GS (2012) A comparison of epidural analgesia and traditional pain management effects on survival and cancer recurrence after colectomy: a population-based study. Anesthesiology 116:797–806

Dave RS, Khalili K (2010) Morphine treatment of human monocyte-derived macrophages induces differential miRNA and protein expression: impact on inflammation and oxidative stress in the central nervous system. J Cell Biochem 110:834–845

Day A, Smith R, Jourdan I, Fawcett W, Scott M, Rockall T (2012) Retrospective analysis of the effect of postoperative analgesia on survival in patients after laparoscopic resection of colorectal cancer. Br J Anaesth 109:185–190

De Oliveira G, Jr AS, Schink JC, Singh DK, Fitzgerald PC, McCarthy RJ (2011) Intraoperative neuraxial anesthesia but not postoperative neuraxial analgesia is associated with increased relapse-free survival in ovarian cancer patients after primary cytoreductive surgery. Reg Anesth Pain Med 36:271–277

Eisenstein TK, Rogers TJ, Meissler JJ Jr, Adler MW, Hilburger ME (1998) Morphine depresses macrophage numbers and function in mouse spleens. Adv Exp Med Biol 437:33–41

Eisenstein TK, Rahim R, Feng P, Thingalaya N, Meissler J (2006) Effects of opioid tolerance and withdrawal on the immune system. J Neuroimmune Pharmacol 1:237–249

Exadaktylos AK, Buggy DJ, Moriarty DC, Mascha E, Sessler DI (2006) Can anesthetic technique for primary breast cancer surgery affect recurrence or metastasis? Anesthesiology 105:660–664

Farooqui M, Geng ZH, Stephenson EJ, Zaveri N, Yee D, Gupta K (2006) Naloxone acts as an antagonist of estrogen receptor activity in MCF-7 cells. Mol Cancer Ther 5:611–620

Fimiani C, Arcuri E, Santoni A, Rialas CM, Bilfinger TV, Peter D, Salzet B, Stefano GB (1999) Mu3 Opiate receptor expression in lung and lung carcinoma: ligand binding and coupling to nitric oxide release. Cancer Lett 146:45–51

Forget P, Tombal B, Scholtes JL, Nzimbala J, Meulders C, Legrand C, Van Cangh P, Cosyns JP, De Kock M (2011) Do intraoperative analgesics influence oncological outcomes after radical prostatectomy for prostate cancer? Eur J Anaesthesiol 28:830–835

Fuggetta MP, Di Francesco P, Falchetti R, Cottarelli A, Rossi L, Tricarico M, Lanzilli G (2005) Effect of morphine on cell-mediated immune responses of human lymphocytes against allogeneic malignant cells. J Exp Clin Cancer Res 24:255–263

Fujioka N, Nguyen J, Chen C, Li Y, Pasrija T, Niehans G, Johnson KN, Gupta V, Kratzke RA, Gupta K (2011) Morphine-induced epidermal growth factor pathway activation in non-small cell lung cancer. Anesth Analg 113:1353–1364

Glattard E, Welters ID, Lavaux T, Muller AH, Laux A, Zhang D, Schmidt AR, Delalande F, Laventie BJ, Dirrig-Grosch S, Colin DA, Van Dorsselaer A, Aunis D, Metz-Boutigue MH, Schneider F, Goumon Y (2010) Endogenous morphine levels are increased in sepsis: a partial implication of neutrophils. PLoS One 5:e8791

Gupta K (2013) Iatrogenic angiogenesis. In: Parat MO (ed) Morphine and metastasis. Springer, Dordrecht

Gupta K, Kshirsagar S, Chang L, Schwartz R, Law PY, Yee D, Hebbel RP (2002) Morphine stimulates angiogenesis by activating proangiogenic and survival-promoting signaling and promotes breast tumor growth. Cancer Res 62:4491–4498

Hashiguchi S, Morisaki H, Kotake Y, Takeda J (2005) Effects of morphine and its metabolites on immune function in advanced cancer patients. J Clin Anesth 17:575–580

Hassan F, Islam S, Tumurkhuu G, Naiki Y, Koide N, Mori I, Yoshida T, Yokochi T (2006) Intracellular expression of toll-like receptor 4 in neuroblastoma cells and their unresponsiveness to lipopolysaccharide. BMC Cancer 6:281

He Y, Wang ZJ (2012) Let-7 microRNAs and opioid tolerance. Front Genet 3:110

He Y, Yang C, Kirkmire CM, Wang ZJ (2010) Regulation of opioid tolerance by let-7 family microRNA targeting the mu opioid receptor. J Neurosci 30:10251–10258

Hoskin PJ, Hanks GW, Aherne GW, Chapman D, Littleton P, Filshie J (1989) The bioavailability and pharmacokinetics of morphine after intravenous, oral and buccal administration in healthy volunteers. Br J Clin Pharmacol 27:499–505

Ishikawa M, Tanno K, Kamo A, Takayanagi Y, Sasaki K (1993) Enhancement of tumor growth by morphine and its possible mechanism in mice. Biol Pharm Bull 16:762–766

Johnson KN, Zaveri N, Gupta K (2013) Interaction of naloxone and estrogen receptor in breast cancer. In: Parat MO (ed) Morphine and metastasis. Springer, Dordrecht

Kasai S, Ikeda K (2011) Pharmacogenomics of the human mu opioid receptor. Pharmacogenomics 12:1305–1320

Klepstad P, Rakvag TT, Kaasa S, Holthe M, Dale O, Borchgrevink PC, Baar C, Vikan T, Krokan HE, Skorpen F (2004) The 118 A>G polymorphism in the human mu opioid receptor gene may increase morphine requirements in patients with pain caused by malignant disease. Acta Anaesthesiol Scand 48:1232–1239

Koodie L, Roy S (2013) Morphine and immunosuppression in the context of tumor growth and metastasis. In: Parat MO (ed) Morphine and metastasis. Springer, Dordrecht

Koodie L, Ramakrishnan S, Roy S (2010) Morphine suppresses tumor angiogenesis through a HIF-1alpha/p38MAPK pathway. Am J Pathol 177:984–997

Kuo CK, Hanioka N, Hoshikawa Y, Oguri K, Yoshimura H (1991) Species difference of site-selective glucuronidation of morphine. J Pharmacobiodyn 14:187–193

Lennon FE, Singleton PA (2013) Opioid regulation of vascular integrity. In: Parat MO (ed) Morphine and metastasis. Springer, Dordrecht

Madbouly KM, Senagore AJ, Delaney CP (2010) Endogenous morphine levels after laparoscopic versus open colectomy. Br J Surg 97:759–764

Martini L, Whistler JL (2007) The role of mu opioid receptor desensitization and endocytosis in morphine tolerance and dependence. Curr Opin Neurobiol 17:556–564

Mathew B, Lennon FE, Siegler J, Mirzapoiazova T, Mambetsariev N, Sammani S, Gerhold LM, LaRiviere PJ, Chen CT, Garcia JGN, Salgia R, Moss J, Singleton PA (2011) The novel role of the mu opioid receptor in lung cancer progression: a laboratory investigation. Anesth Analg 112:558–567

Molteni M, Marabella D, Orlandi C, Rossetti C (2006) Melanoma cell lines are responsive in vitro to lipopolysaccharide and express TLR-4. Cancer Lett 235:75–83

Muller A, Glattard E, Taleb O, Kemmel V, Laux A, Miehe M, Delalande F, Roussel G, Van Dorsselaer A, Metz-Boutigue MH, Aunis D, Goumon Y (2008) Endogenous morphine in SH-SY5Y cells and the mouse cerebellum. PLoS One 3:e1641

Munjal ID, Minna JD, Manneckjee R, Bieck P, Spector S (1995) Possible role of endogenous morphine and codeine on growth regulation of lung tissue. Life Sci 57:517–521

Myles PS, Peyton P, Silbert B, Hunt J, Rigg JR, Sessler DI (2011) Perioperative epidural analgesia for major abdominal surgery for cancer and recurrence-free survival: randomised trial. BMJ 342:d1491
Nagano E, Yamada H, Oguri K (2000) Characteristic glucuronidation pattern of physiologic concentration of morphine in rat brain. Life Sci 67:2453–2464
Osborne R, Joel S, Trew D, Slevin M (1988) Analgesic activity of morphine-6-glucuronide. Lancet 331:828
Osborne R, Joel S, Trew D, Slevin M (1990) Morphine and metabolite behavior after different routes of morphine administration: demonstration of the importance of the active metabolite morphine-6-glucuronide. Clin Pharmacol Ther 47:12–19
Page GG, Ben-Eliyahu S, Yirmiya R, Liebeskind JC (1993) Morphine attenuates surgery-induced enhancement of metastatic colonization in rats. Pain 54:21–28
Page GG, Ben-Eliyahu S, Liebeskind JC (1994) The role of LGL/NK cells in surgery-induced promotion of metastasis and its attenuation by morphine. Brain Behav Immun 8:241–250
Page GG, McDonald JS, Ben-Eliyahu S (1998) Pre-operative versus postoperative administration of morphine: impact on the neuroendocrine, behavioural, and metastatic-enhancing effects of surgery. Br J Anaesth 81:216–223
Page GG, Blakely WP, Ben-Eliyahu S (2001) Evidence that postoperative pain is a mediator of the tumor-promoting effects of surgery in rats. Pain 90:191–199
Poeaknapo C, Schmidt J, Brandsch M, Drager B, Zenk MH (2004) Endogenous formation of morphine in human cells. Proc Natl Acad Sci USA 101:14091–14096
Popping DM, Wenk M, Schug SA (2013) Anaesthetic and pain management technique in long term cancer outcome – benefits of regional anaesthesia and analgesia in the context of cancer surgery. In: Parat MO (ed) Morphine and metastasis. Springer, Dordrecht
Sasamura T, Nakamura S, Iida Y, Fujii H, Murata J, Saiki I, Nojima H, Kuraishi Y (2002) Morphine analgesia suppresses tumor growth and metastasis in a mouse model of cancer pain produced by orthotopic tumor inoculation. Eur J Pharmacol 441:185–191
Schoof CR, Botelho EL, Izzotti A, Vasques LR (2012) MicroRNAs in cancer treatment and prognosis. Am J Cancer Res 2:414–433
Sessler DI, Ben-Eliyahu S, Mascha EJ, Parat MO, Buggy DJ (2008) Can regional analgesia reduce the risk of recurrence after breast cancer? Methodology of a multicenter randomized trial. Contemp Clin Trials 29:517–526
Shanahan H, Parat MO, Buggy DJ (2013) Could opioids affect cancer recurrence or metastases? Current experimental and translational evidence. In: Parat MO (ed) Morphine and metastasis. Springer, Dordrecht
Shigeta Y, Kasai S, Han W, Hata H, Nishi A, Takamatsu Y, Hagino Y, Yamamoto H, Koide T, Shiroishi T, Kasai K, Tsunashima K, Kato N, Ikeda K (2008) Association of morphine-induced antinociception with variations in the 5′ flanking and 3′ untranslated regions of the mu opioid receptor gene in 10 inbred mouse strains. Pharmacogenet Genomics 18:927–936
Shilling AM, Tiouririne M (2013) Perioperative morphine and cancer recurrence. In: Parat MO (ed) Morphine and metastasis. Springer, Dordrecht
Shimomura K, Kamata O, Ueki S, Ida S, Oguri K, Yoshimura H, Tsukamoto H (1971) Analgesic effect of morphine glucuronides. Tohoku J Exp Med 105:45–52
Sia AT, Lim Y, Lim EC, Goh RW, Law HY, Landau R, Teo YY, Tan EC (2008) A118G single nucleotide polymorphism of human mu-opioid receptor gene influences pain perception and patient-controlled intravenous morphine consumption after intrathecal morphine for postcesarean analgesia. Anesthesiology 109:520–526
Singleton PA, Lingen MW, Fekete MJ, Garcia JGN, Moss J (2006) Methylnaltrexone inhibits opiate and VEGF-induced angiogenesis: role of receptor transactivation. Microvasc Res 72:3–11
Stefano GB, Hartman A, Bilfinger TV, Magazine HI, Liu Y, Casares F, Goligorsky MS (1995) Presence of the mu3 opiate receptor in endothelial cells: coupling to nitric oxide production and vasodilation. J Biol Chem 270:30290–30293
Stefano GB, Ptacek R, Kuzelova H, Kream RM (2012) Endogenous morphine: up-to-date review (2011). Folia Biol (Praha) 58:49–56

Tang XY, Zhu YQ, Wei B, Wang H (2010) Expression and functional research of TLR4 in human colon carcinoma. Am J Med Sci 339:319–326

Thornton JE, Gregory RI (2012) How does Lin28 let-7 control development and disease? Trends Cell Biol. doi:10.1016/j.tcb.2012.06.001

Tsui BC, Rashiq S, Schopflocher D, Murtha A, Broemling S, Pillay J, Finucane BT (2010) Epidural anesthesia and cancer recurrence rates after radical prostatectomy. Can J Anaesth 57:107–112

Wang S, Li Y, Liu XD, Zhao CX, Yang KQ (2012a) Polymorphism of A118G in mu-opioid receptor gene is associated with risk of esophageal squamous cell carcinoma in a Chinese population. Int J Clin Oncol. doi:10.1007/s10147-012-0441-5

Wang X, Cao L, Wang Y, Wang X, Liu N, You Y (2012b) Regulation of let-7 and its target oncogenes (review). Oncol Lett 3:955–960

Wang X, Loram LC, Ramos K, de Jesus AJ, Thomas J, Cheng K, Reddy A, Somogyi AA, Hutchinson MR, Watkins LR, Yin H (2012c) Morphine activates neuroinflammation in a manner parallel to endotoxin. Proc Natl Acad Sci USA 109:6325–6330

Wang Y, Barker K, Shi S, Diaz M, Mo B, Gutstein HB (2012d) Blockade of PDGFR-[beta] activation eliminates morphine analgesic tolerance. Nat Med 18:385–387

Wuethrich PY, Hsu Schmitz SF, Kessler TM, Thalmann GN, Studer UE, Stueber F, Burkhard FC (2010) Potential influence of the anesthetic technique used during open radical prostatectomy on prostate cancer-related outcome: a retrospective study. Anesthesiology 113:570–576

Yeager MP, Colacchio TA (1991) Effect of morphine on growth of metastatic colon cancer in vivo. Arch Surg 126:454–456

Yoshida S, Ohta J, Yamasaki K, Kamei H, Harada Y, Yahara T, Kaibara A, Ozaki K, Tajiri T, Shirouzu K (2000) Effect of surgical stress on endogenous morphine and cytokine levels in the plasma after laparoscopic or open cholecystectomy. Surg Endosc 14:137–140

Yuan CS, Foss JF, O'Connor M, Toledano A, Roizen MF, Moss J (1996) Methylnaltrexone prevents morphine-induced delay in oral-cecal transit time without affecting analgesia: a double-blind randomized placebo-controlled trial. Clin Pharmacol Ther 59:469–475

Zheng H, Zeng Y, Zhang X, Chu J, Loh HH, Law PY (2010) Mu-opioid receptor agonists differentially regulate the expression of miR-190 and NeuroD. Mol Pharmacol 77:102–109

Zhu W, Cadet P, Baggerman G, Mantione KJ, Stefano GB (2005) Human white blood cells synthesize morphine: CYP2D6 modulation. J Immunol 175:7357–7362

# Chapter 2
# Interaction of Naloxone and Estrogen Receptor in Breast Cancer

**Katherine N.H. Johnson, Nurulain Zaveri, and Kalpna Gupta**

**Abstract** Majority of breast cancers are estrogen receptor (ER) positive. Due to resistance to known ER-based therapies, novel treatment targets and drugs are required to effectively treat ER-positive breast cancer. Opioids are often used to treat pain in breast cancer and promote tumor growth and metastases in rodent studies. Opioid receptor (OR) antagonists, such as naloxone, naltrexone and methylnaltrexone inhibit cancer progression and metastases. All three antagonists share structural similarities with the estrogen, 17β-estradiol (E2), and are therefore capable of binding to ER. Naloxone inhibits E2-induced human MCF-7 breast cancer cell proliferation and MAPK/ERK signaling. Additionally, naloxone also attenuates the activation of membrane bound/cytoplasmic ER and phosphorylation of the epidermal growth factor receptor. Naloxone blocks the E2-induced ER activation by precluding its binding to the co-activator and by directly competing with E2 for binding to ER. In addition to these direct interactions with ER, naloxone prevents the cross-talk of ER with mu opioid receptor (MOR), suggesting that activation of MOR may contribute to E2-induced ER activation. Since naloxone and structurally similar OR antagonists inhibit cancer progression and metastases, OR antagonists can be potentially developed for breast cancer treatment.

**Keywords** Angiogenesis • Breast cancer • EGF receptor • Estrogen receptor • G protein coupled receptors • Methylnaltrexone • Naloxone • Naltrexone • Opioid receptor • Therapy

---

K.N.H. Johnson • K. Gupta, Ph.D. (✉)
Department of Medicine – Hematology, Oncology and Transplantation and Vascular Biology Center, University of Minnesota, Mayo Mail Code 480, 420 Delaware Street SE, Minneapolis, MN 55455, USA
e-mail: gupta014@umn.edu

N. Zaveri, Ph.D.
Astraea Therapeutics, LLC, 320 Logue Avenue, Suite 142, Mountain View, CA 94043, USA
e-mail: nurulain@astraeatherapeutics.com

M.-O. Parat (ed.), *Morphine and Metastasis*, DOI 10.1007/978-94-007-5678-6_2, 

## Abbreviations

| | |
|---|---|
| E2 | 17β-estradiol |
| AF1 | activation-function 1 |
| AF2 | activation-function 2 |
| AI | aromatase inhibitor |
| cAMP | cyclic adenosine monophosphate |
| EGFR | epidermal growth factor receptor |
| ER | estrogen receptor |
| ERE | estrogen response element |
| Gi-GPCRs | inhibitory regulated-G protein coupled receptors |
| LBD | ligand-binding domain |
| MNTX | methylnaltrexone |
| MAPK/ERK | mitogen activated protein kinase/extracellular signal-regulated kinase |
| Nal | naloxone |
| NTX | naltrexone |
| NOP | nociceptin/orphanin FQ receptor |
| OR | opioid receptor |
| PI3K | phosphatidylinositol 3-kinase |
| Akt | protein kinase B |
| SERMs | selective ER modulators |
| VEGFR2 | vascular endothelial growth factor receptor 2 |
| DOR | δ opioid receptor |
| KOR | κ opioid receptor |
| MOR | μ opioid receptor |

## 2.1 Interaction of Naloxone and Estrogen Receptor in Breast Cancer

In the developed world breast cancer is the most common malignancy amongst women. It is estimated that in the United States (US) alone, about 12% of women, which amounts to one out of eight women, will develop invasive breast cancer in their life-time (www.breastcancer.org). An alarming number of new cases of invasive and non-invasive breast cancer (230,480 and 57,650, respectively) were to be diagnosed in women and 39,520 women were expected to die of breast cancer in 2011 in the US. In spite of a slow decline in the breast cancer incidence, (about 2%) due to increased awareness, early detection and treatment, breast cancer remains the second most common malignancy in women in the US. About 80% of breast cancers are estrogen-receptor positive. Therefore, strategies to attenuate estrogen receptor (ER) activity are critical to cure breast cancer.

## 2.2 Role of Estrogen Receptor

The ER is a member of the nuclear steroid-hormone receptor superfamily (Mangelsdorf et al. 1995; Hall et al. 2001). The two isoforms of ER, ERα and ERβ, have a high degree of homology, particularly in their ligand and DNA binding domains and exhibit the characteristic features common to intracellular nuclear receptors (Hall et al. 2001). ERα- and ERβ-knockout mice display different phenotypes. Female ERα-knockout mice show complete estrogen insensitivity in the reproductive organs, and have stunted mammary glandsin addition to other phenotypic changes, whereas, female ERβ-knockout mice have limited ovarian function (Lubahn et al. 1993; Krege et al. 1998; Dupont et al. 2000; Korach et al. 2003). Both isoforms play a critical role in the normal and malignant biology of the breast, where, ERα is the predominant form in neoplastic breast epithelium, while ERβ is more common in normal breast tissue (Khan et al. 1994; Hall et al. 2001). It is suggested that ERβ may regulate ERα activation, by decreasing cellular sensitivity to estrogens (Hall and McDonnell 1999).

ERα-dependent breast cancer progression has been a subject of intense investigation to develop targeted therapies. About one third of breast cancers are ERα-negative and difficult to treat, but about 65% are ER-positive (Howe and Brown 2011). Several ERα-based drugs are suggested to have a preventive effect on breast cancer in women at moderate- to high-risk of developing breast cancer based on a large phase III clinical trial (Cuzick et al. 2011; Vogel et al. 2010). Drugs tested included the aromatase inhibitor (AI), exemestane and selective ER modulators (SERMs), tamoxifen, raloxifene and lasofoxifene. These drugs reduce the risk of developing breast cancer and are also used to treat ERα-positive breast cancer. In spite of the promising effect of these therapies, patients with breast cancer develop resistance to therapy. Epidermal growth factor receptor family, ErbB family, which includes the epidermal growth factor receptor (EGFR), has been suggested to play an important role in development of resistance to hormonal therapy (Massarweh et al. 2008; Arpino et al. 2004; Emde et al. 2011). Thus a sub-set of ER-positive breast cancer's therapeutic outcomes are challenged by activation of alternative growth factor signaling pathways.

## 2.3 Mechanism of Action of ER

ERs display the characteristic features of nuclear hormone receptors. Structurally, ERα acts in a ligand-dependent as well as ligand-independent way (Gronemeyer et al. 2004; Nilsson et al. 2011). The amino terminal activation-function 1 (AF1) activates ligand-independent transcription and the carboxy terminal, activation-function 2 (AF 2) region consists of a multifunctional ligand-binding domain (LBD). The central region consists of the DNA-binding domain, which binds to the specific sequence of DNA on the estrogen response element (ERE) for transcriptional activation. The transcriptional activity of ER further depends upon activating and repressing co-regulators in the nucleus.

ERα exists in an inactive form in the cytoplasm and nucleus of the cell. Ligand binding induces a conformational change resulting in homodimerization and nuclear translocation, followed by binding to the ERE and transcriptional activation (Nilsson et al. 2011). In addition to the classical activation by specific ligands, cytoplasmic ERs are phosphorylated by activated growth factor receptors, such as EGFR. In turn, activated cytoplasmic ERs stimulate mitogen activated protein kinase/extracellular signal-regulated kinase (MAPK/ERK) and phosphatidylinositol 3-kinase (PI3K)-protein kinase B (Akt) phosphorylation directly as well as by a cross talk with inhibitory regulated-G protein coupled receptors (Gi-GPCRs) (Hammes and Levin 2007; Wu et al. 2011). However, cytoplasmic activation of the ERs does not promote breast cancer growth, but stimulates endothelial cell-specific activities. In a tumor microenvironment, activated growth factor receptors and GPCRs may therefore further promote ER-induced cell survival and proliferation in breast cancer, by contributing to increased angiogenesis and perhaps increased resistance to hormonal therapy.

## 2.4 Opioid Receptors

Gi-GPCR family includes opioid receptors (OR). The significance of OR activity is two-fold in cancer biology because: (1) OR agonists such as morphine are often used to treat severe pain in cancer and (2) opioid-induced cell survival and proliferation may contribute to cancer progression and metastases directly and by promoting angiogenesis (Gupta et al. 2002, 2007; Stephenson and Gupta 2006; Farooqui et al. 2007; Singleton et al. 2006).

There are four different classes of classical ORs –μ, δ, κ (MOR, DOR, and KOR, respectively) and nociceptin/orphanin FQ receptor (NOP) (Finley et al. 2008; Gupta et al. 2007; Stephenson and Gupta 2006). These receptors are coupled to Gi/Go type of G-protein and inhibit adenyl cyclase activity resulting in a decrease in the basal production of cyclic adenosine monophosphate (cAMP). However, chronic activation of ORs may lead to superactivation of adenyl cyclase and increased cAMP (Gupta et al. 2007). Depending upon its binding affinity each opioid is a selective agonist for a specific receptor, whereas, Naloxone (Nal) is a non-selective antagonist.

## 2.5 Possible Role of Naloxone in Cancer

Opioid receptor antagonists, such as Nal and Naltrexone (NTX), were shown to inhibit the growth of neuroblastoma and mammary tumors in vivo, almost three decades ago (Aylsworth et al. 1979; Zagon and McLaughlin 1983b; Tsunashima 1982).

These observations support the antitumor activity of OR antagonists, but raise the possibility that these antagonists may attenuate the analgesic ability of endogenous opioids and exogenously administered opioid analgesic drugs. However, more recent studies suggest an anti-nociceptive effect of a low dose of naloxone by itself and/or co-administered with opioids (Lunzer et al. 2007; Power 2011).

The MCF-7 cell line is a widely studied human breast cancer tumor model that is estrogen dependent. Several studies with MCF-7 cells suggest the modulatory effects of opioids and their receptor(s) on estrogen and its receptor(s) and vice versa (Table 2.1) (Cadet et al. 2002; Panagiotou et al. 1998; Sinchak and Micevych 2001). In earlier studies, however, opioid-induced cell proliferation was Nal-insensitive in vitro, yet Nal potently inhibited tumor growth in vivo (Gupta et al. 2002; Tegeder et al. 2003; Maneckjee and Minna 1992; Kugawa et al. 1998; Hatzoglou et al. 1996a; b). We found that morphine stimulated angiogenesis and human MCF-7 breast cancer cell tumor xenografts in nude mice, whereas, Nal inhibited tumor growth in this model (Gupta et al. 2002). Intriguingly, more recent studies from our laboratory showed that 17 β-estradiol (E2)-induced MCF-7 breast cancer cell proliferation was inhibited by 100 nM Nal, but not by morphine (Farooqui et al. 2006). Together, these observations suggest an interaction of Nal with the E2-stimulated pathways and/or antagonism of constitutively activated ORs in MCF-7 cells. Thus, morphine appears to promote cancer growth by promoting angiogenesis, and Nal attenuates breast cancer progression by acting directly on the cancer cells.

## 2.6 Structural Similarity Between ER Agonists/ER Antagonists and OR Antagonists

We observed that the phenolic hydroxyl group required for the binding of ER ligands to ER is also present in Nal (Farooqui et al. 2006; Fig. 2.1). The phenolic hydroxyl group is a common feature of several OR antagonists including NTX and methylnaltrexone (MNTX). Superimposition of energy-minimized conformations of E2 (magenta), Nal (cyan), and MNTX (yellow), show the overlap of the phenolic hydroxy-bearing aromatic ring (solid white arrow) of all the compounds (Fig. 2.1a). The N-allyl and cyclopropylmethyl substituents of Nal and MNTX respectively, occupy the same region in space as the D-ring of the steroidal E2 (Fig. 2.1a). Superimposition of energy-minimized conformations of E2 (green), NTX (yellow), MNTX (magenta) and 4-hydroxytamoxifen (cyan), depict the overlap of the phenolic hydroxy-bearing aromatic ring (solid red arrow) (Fig. 2.1b). The N-substitution of NTX and MNTX occupies the same region of space as the D-ring of E2 (green arrow), and may be responsible for their action as antagonists of ER. This conclusion is corroborated by the observations that Nal inhibits the binding of E2 to ERα in vitro (Farooqui et al. 2006).

**Table 2.1** Effects of opioid receptor antagonists on cancer model systems

| Opioid receptor antagonist | Dose/route of administration | Model system | Outcome | Reference |
|---|---|---|---|---|
| *Naloxone* | 0.356 and 0.72 mg/kg/day s.c. for the first and second week, respectively | Human MCF-7 breast cancer cell xenograft in athymic nude mice | Inhibition of tumor growth and angiogenesis; and inhibition of morphine-induced tumor growth and angiogenesis | Gupta et al. (2002) |
| | 100 nmol/L | Human MCF-7 breast cancer cell line | Inhibits basal and 17-β estradiol-induced proliferation and MAPK/ERK phosphorylation | Farooqui et al. (2006) |
| | 100 nM | Human non-small cell lung cancer cell line, H2009 | Naloxone inhibits MS and EGF induced phosphorylation of EGFR, MAPK/ERK, and Akt and cellular proliferation and invasion | Fujioka et al. (2011) |
| | 1 mM for 6 h | Human ovarian cancer cell line, SKOV-3 | Naloxone inhibited cell number by 28% | Donahue et al. (2011b) |
| | 1 μM for 6 h | Human ovarian cancer cell line, SKOV-3 | Naloxone did not affect cell number | Donahue et al. (2011b) |
| | 1 μM | Human ovarian cancer cell lines, OVCAR-3, SKOV-3 | Naloxone in the absence or presence of 1 μM OGF did not affect ovarian cancer cell proliferation | Donahue et al. (2009) |
| | 100 nmol/L | Human MCF-7 breast cancer cell line | Naloxone blocks opioid induced down regulation of MOR | Gach et al. (2008) |
| | 100 nmol/L | Human MCF-7 breast cancer cell line | Naloxone increased MOR mRNA expression by 20% and protein expression by 68% | Gach et al. (2008) |
| | 100 nmol/L | Human MCF-7 breast cancer cell line | Naloxone administration stimulated the complex formation of NF-κB and AP-1 with the MOR promoter | Gach et al. (2008) |
| *Naltrexone* | 75 mg/kg/day in diet | 7,12-dimethylbenz(a) anthracene (DMBA)-induced rat mammary tumors | Naltrexone inhibited tumor multiplicity by 40% when administered at tumor initiation, 73% at tumor promotion, and 70% when administered during initiation and promotion | Koo et al. (1996) |

| | | | | |
|---|---|---|---|---|
| | 0.1 mg/kg/i.p. | Human ovarian cancer cell line SKOV-3 was injected in athymic nu/nu mice and tumors nodules on the surface of liver, stomach, spleen and mesentery/intestine were analyzed | Naltrexone reduced tumor nodules and weight by inhibiting proliferation and angiogenesis | Donahue et al. (2011b) |
| | $10^{-5}$ M | Human ovarian cancer cell line, SKOV-3 | Short-term (6 h) Naltrexone treatment inhibited but continuous exposure increased cell proliferation. Naltrexone in conjunction with taxol or cisplatin reduced cell proliferation as compared to either treatment alone | Donahue et al. (2011a) |
| | $10^{-5}$ M short term or continuous exposure of cells in vitro | Multiple human cancer cell lines SKOV-3, OVCAR-3, SCC-1, MiaPaCa-2, HCT-1 | Inhibition of proliferation by sort-term (6 h) treatment via opioid growth factor receptor | Donahue et al. (2011a) |
| | 100 mg given orally every other day | Patients with untreatable metastatic solid tumors | Naltrexone amplifies lymphocytosis induced by IL-2 and melatonin to enhance their immunotherapeutic ability | Lissoni et al. (2002) |
| | $10^{-6}$ M | Various cancer cell lines; CAL 27, MIA PaCa-2, BxPC-3, HT-29, HCT 116, SKOV-3, OVCAR-3, H226, A549, DU 145, PC-3, SK-HEP, Hep G2, Ht-1080, S-ES-1, SW 1088, U-87 MG, U251, SK-N-SH, **MDA-MB-231**, **MCF7**, K-562, AGS, U266, MES-SA, Caki-2, Flo-1, SCC-1, UACC903, 1205 LU, KAT-18 | Increased cancer cell proliferation | Zagon et al. (2009) |

(continued)

Table 2.1 (continued)

| Opioid receptor antagonist | Dose/route of administration | Model system | Outcome | Reference |
|---|---|---|---|---|
| | 0.1 mg/kg daily, tri-weekly, or weekly | Human squamous cell carcinoma cell line SCC-1 xenografted in BALB/c athymic nude mice | Increased latency, decreased tumor volume, weight and BrdU incorporation | McLaughlin and Zagon (2012) |
| | 1 μM | OVCAR-3, SKOV-3 | Naltrexone increased ovarian cancer cell proliferation | Donahue et al. (2009) |
| | 4.5 mg orally at bedtime | Pancreatic cancer with metastasis | Naltrexone given with α-lipoic acid attenuated pancreatic tumor and metastasis | Berkson et al. (2009) |
| *Methylnaltrexone* | 10 and 100 nM | Lewis Lung Carcinoma (LLC) | Methylnaltrexone significantly reduced LLC cellular invasion | Mathew et al. (2011) |
| | 10 mg/kg/day, s.c. | Xenograft Lewis lung carcinoma r mouse model | Methylnaltrexone significantly reduced tumor volume, tumor weight and lung metastasis | Mathew et al. (2011) |
| | 100 nM | Human pulmonary vein microvascular endothelial cells (HPMVEC) | Methylnaltrexone lowered the $IC_{50}$ of 5-FU from 5 μmol/L to 7 nmol/L and inhibited Src and Akt activation via MOR | Singleton et al. (2008) |
| | 50 ng/mL | HPMVEC | Methylnaltrexone lowered the $IC_{50}$ of bevacizumab from 25 to 6 ng/mL and inhibited Src and Akt activation via MOR | Singleton et al. (2008) |
| | 0.1–500 nM | HPMVEC | Methylnaltrexone alone and in conjunction with mTOR inhibitors reduced VEGF-induced endothelial proliferation and angiogenesis | Singleton et al. (2010) |
| | 100 nM | C57BL6 Mice | Methylnaltrexone alone and in conjunction with mTOR inhibitors reduced angiogenesis | Singleton et al. (2010) |
| | 0.1 μM | Human dermal microvascular endothelial cells | Inhibition of VEGF-induced migration, angiogenesis and RhoA activation | Singleton et al. (2006) |

Abbreviations used: *MOR* mu opioid receptor, *LLC* Lewis lung carcinoma, *HPMVEC* Human pulmonary vein microvascular endothelial cells, *i.p.* intraperitoneally, *s.c.* subcutaneously

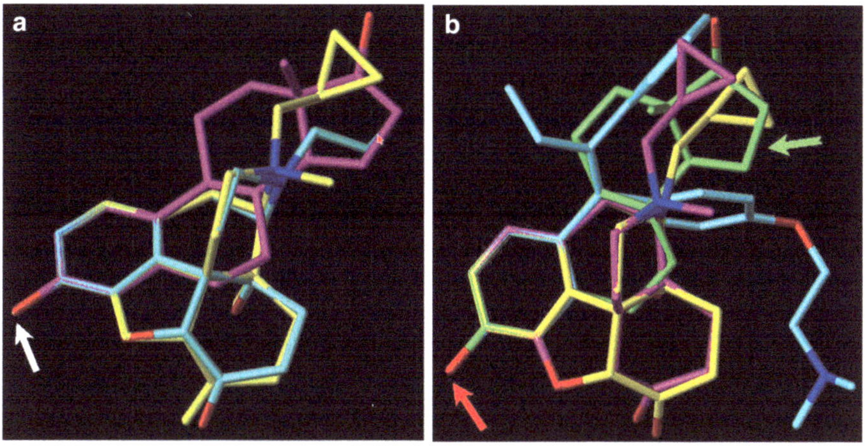


**Fig. 2.1** Structural similarities between estrogen and opioid receptor antagonists, naloxone, naltrexone and methylnaltrexone. (**a**) Superimposition of energy-minimized structures of E2 (*magenta*), Nal (*cyan*), and MNTX (*yellow*). (**b**) Superimposition of energy-minimized conformations of E2 (*green*), NTX (*yellow*), MNTX (*magenta*) and 4-hydroxytamoxifen (*cyan*)

## 2.7 Inhibition of Breast Cancer Growth by Naloxone

Nal at 1.5 mg/kg/day and 10–30 mg/kg/day reduces tumor volume by ~25–30% in nude mice xenografted with MCF-7 human breast cancer cells, compared to controls (Gupta et al. 2002; Tegeder et al. 2003). Nal also antagonizes the genomic and non-genomic activity of ERα in MCF-7cells (Farooqui et al. 2006). It is important to antagonize ERα activity since most human breast tumors are ERα-positive and respond to estrogen/hormonal therapy, but often develop resistance to therapy. Due to structural similarities with ERα agonists and antagonists, Nal binds to ERα and modulates its activity directly. Nal inhibits E2-induced MAPK/ERK phosphorylation and MCF7 cell proliferation by 65%. Nal directly inhibits the E2-induced activation of ERα by binding to the nuclear ERα, and inhibits E2-induced down-regulation of ERα mRNA, required for receptor re-activation. Moreover, Nal inhibits the non-genomic activity of ERα by inhibiting the binding of E2 to the plasma membrane. In the presence of Nal, ERα associates with MOR only when activated with E2, suggesting the possibility of MOR-induced transactivation of ER (Farooqui et al. 2006).

Nal and NTX are structurally similar OR antagonists that non-selectively bind all three classical ORs and antagonize the analgesic activity of opioids. NTX inhibited neuroblastoma growth at low doses (0.1mg/kg), but stimulated it at high doses (10mg/kg) in both immunodeficient and immunocompetent mice. NTX (0.1 mg/kg) increased tumor latency to 98%, increased survival by 36%, but also blocked morphine-induced analgesia for 4–6 h compared to controls (Zagon and McLaughlin 1983a, b, 1987). In contrast, 10 mg/kg NTX had the opposite effect on tumor incidence, latency, survival and metastasis, and blocked morphine-induced analgesia for 24 h. NTX (75 mg/kg diet) also inhibited the initiation (I), progression (P), and I+P phase of DMBA-induced rat mammary tumors by 27, 60, and 45%, respectively (Koo et al. 1996) and reduced tumor multiplicity by 40, 73, and 70%, respectively. These effects of Nal and NTX support the hypothesis that OR antogonists structurally similar to ERα could be used to treat and inhibit human cancer growth.

Another OR antagonist, MNTX is a quaternary derivative of NTX, with a methyl group attached to the amine of NTX, has a greater polarity, lower lipid solubility and structural similarity to Nal as described above (Moss and Rosow 2008). Unlike Nal and NTX, MNTX is MOR-selective and does not cross the blood–brain barrier. Therefore MNTX does not antagonize opioid analgesia. MNTX inhibits MOR-mediated vascular endothelial growth factor receptor 2 (VEGFR2) crosstalk, potentiates the apoptotic effect of mTOR inhibitors, inhibits angiogenesis and inhibits lung cancer progression and metastasis (Lennon et al. 2012; Mathew et al. 2011; Singleton et al. 2006, 2010). Table 2.1 lists the effects of OR antagonists on a variety of human endothelial and cancer cells, rodent models of cancer and human cancer. Collectively, the antagonism of MOR and inhibition of cancer growth and angiogenesis by the structurally similar OR antagonists argue for their potential in cancer therapeutics.

## 2.8 OR Antagonism May Uncouple Growth Factor Receptor Signaling Pathways

MOR also transactivates EGFR (Belcheva et al. 2001; Fujioka et al. 2011). Morphine stimulates MAPK/ERK phosphorylation in endothelial, breast cancer and lung cancer cells via MOR (Singleton et al. 2006; Gupta et al. 2002; Chen et al. 2006; Mathew et al. 2011; Fujioka et al. 2011). Activation of MAPK/ERK and EGFR activates ERα and may even confer tamoxifen (TAM) resistance (Gururaj et al. 2006; Kato et al. 1995; Ring and Dowsett 2004). Higher levels of met-enkephalin were observed in the plasma of women with breast cancer compared to age-matched controls ($171 \pm 190$ in cancer vs. $109 \pm 79$ in controls) (Kajdaniuk et al. 2000). Increased endogenous opioids may lead to constitutive activation of MOR, which may contribute to the activation of ERα signaling and perhaps ineffectiveness of ERα based hormonal therapy. It is therefore likely that co-administration of Nal and Nal-like antagonists of ORs may increase the therapeutic efficacy of hormonal therapy.

## 2.9 Translational Significance of Naloxone/OR Antagonism in Cancer Therapy

Recent studies demonstrate that OR antagonists such as MNTX, which is structurally similar to Nal can inhibit both endothelial and tumor cell proliferation. Therefore, we propose that Nal and Nal-like OR antagonists may attenuate tumor growth by inhibiting

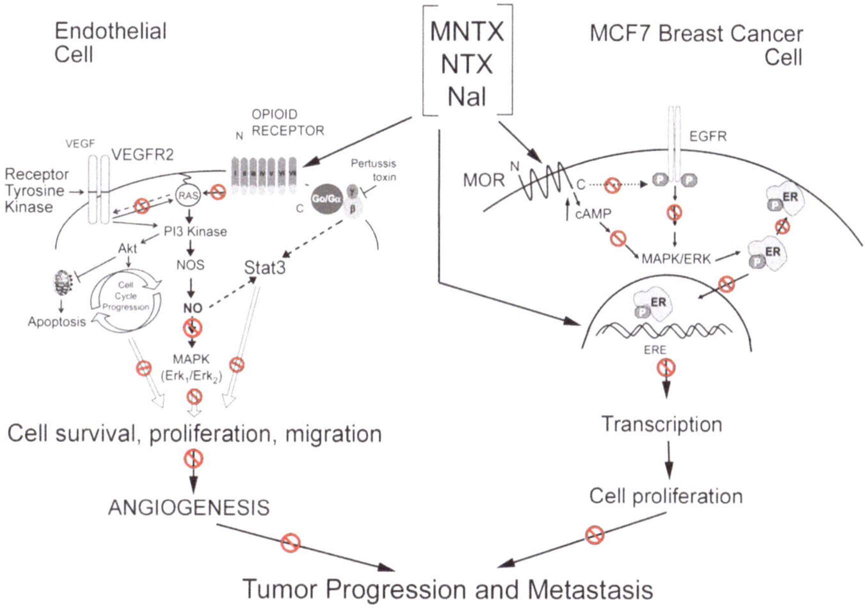


**Fig. 2.2** Proposed model of opioid receptor antagonist(s)-mediated inhibition of breast cancer growth and metastases. Mu opioid receptor transactivates VEGFR2 in endothelium and EGFR and ERα in breast cancer cells. In addition, MOR directly activates angiogenic and growth promoting signaling by activating MAPK/ERK and Stat3 pathway in endothelium. Opioid receptor antagonists, naloxone, naltrexone and methylnaltrexone can inhibit these mitogenic activities of MOR and block cell proliferation. These antagonists can also inhibit the genomic and non-genomic activity of ERα and attenuate estrogen-induced breast cancer cell proliferation (Abbreviations: *VEGF* vascular endothelial cell growth factor, *VEGFR$_2$* VEGF receptor$_2$/Flk1/KDR, *MNTX* methylnaltrexone, *NTX* naltrexone, *Nal*, naloxone; *MOR* mu opioid receptor, *EGFR* epidermal growth factor receptor, *NO* nitric oxide, *ER* estrogen receptor, *ERE* estrogen response element)

pro-angiogenic signaling in endothelium; and by inhibiting estrogen-dependent and -independent breast cancer cell proliferation (Fig. 2.2). Nal/NTX/MNTX will block the OR-mediated transactivation of VEGFR2 signaling that is critical to the promotion of angiogenesis. In breast cancer cells, Nal/NTX/MNTX may inhibit (stop signs) the MOR-dependent EGFR and MAPK/ERK signaling which orchestrates resistance to hormonal therapy, as well as directly antagonizes ERα activity, thereby preventing resistance to therapy and inhibiting breast cancer progression. Since metastasis is dependent upon angiogenesis, the anti-angiogenic effect of OR antagonists may even impair metastases. Together, the OR-dependent and independent effect of Nal in breast cancer, support the development of novel Nal-like drugs for cancer therapy.

**Acknowledgements** The authors thank Ms Carol Taubert for manuscript preparation and figures. This work was supported by National Institutes of Health Grant numbers CA109582, HL068802 and HL103733.

## References

Arpino G, Green SJ, Allred DC, Lew D, Martino S, Osborne CK, Elledge RM (2004) Her-2 amplification, her-1 expression, and tamoxifen response in estrogen receptor-positive metastatic breast cancer: a southwest oncology group study. Clin Cancer Res 10:5670–5676. doi:10.1158/1078-0432.CCR-04-011010/17/5670 [pii]

Aylsworth CF, Hodson CA, Meites J (1979) Opiate antagonists can inhibit mammary tumor growth in rats. Proc Soc Exp Biol Med 161:18–20

Belcheva MM, Szucs M, Wang D, Sadee W, Coscia CJ (2001) Mu-opioid receptor-mediated erk activation involves calmodulin-dependent epidermal growth factor receptor transactivation. J Biol Chem 276:33847–33853

Berkson BM, Rubin DM, Berkson AJ (2009) Revisiting the ala/n (alpha-lipoic acid/low-dose naltrexone) protocol for people with metastatic and nonmetastatic pancreatic cancer: a report of 3 new cases. Integr Cancer Ther 8:416–422. doi:8/4/416 [pii]10.1177/1534735409352082

Cadet P, Mantione K, Bilfinger TV, Stefano GB (2002) Morphine down regulates human vascular tissue estrogen receptor expression determined by real-time RT-PCR. Neuro Endocrinol Lett 23:95–100. doi:NEL230202A01 [pii]

Chen C, Farooqui M, Gupta K (2006) Morphine stimulates vascular endothelial growth factor-like signaling in mouse retinal endothelial cells. Curr Neurovasc Res 3:171–180

Cuzick J, DeCensi A, Arun B, Brown PH, Castiglione M, Dunn B, Forbes JF, Glaus A, Howell A, von Minckwitz G, Vogel V, Zwierzina H (2011) Preventive therapy for breast cancer: a consensus statement. Lancet Oncol 12:496–503. doi:S1470-2045(11)70030-4 [pii]10.1016/S1470-2045(11)70030-4

Donahue RN, McLaughlin PJ, Zagon IS (2009) Cell proliferation of human ovarian cancer is regulated by the opioid growth factor-opioid growth factor receptor axis. Am J Physiol Regul Integr Comp Physiol 296:R1716–R1725

Donahue RN, McLaughlin PJ, Zagon IS (2011a) Low-dose naltrexone targets the opioid growth factor-opioid growth factor receptor pathway to inhibit cell proliferation: mechanistic evidence from a tissue culture model. Exp Biol Med (Maywood) 236:1036–1050. doi:ebm.2011.011121 [pii]10.1258/ebm.2011.011121

Donahue RN, McLaughlin PJ, Zagon IS (2011b) The opioid growth factor (OGF) and low dose naltrexone (LDN) suppress human ovarian cancer progression in mice. Gynecol Oncol 122:382–388. doi:S0090-8258(11)00270-8 [pii]10.1016/j.ygyno.2011.04.009

Dupont S, Krust A, Gansmuller A, Dierich A, Chambon P, Mark M (2000) Effect of single and compound knockouts of estrogen receptors alpha (eralpha) and beta (erbeta) on mouse reproductive phenotypes. Development 127:4277–4291

Emde A, Mahlknecht G, Maslak K, Ribba B, Sela M, Possinger K, Yarden Y (2011) Simultaneous inhibition of estrogen receptor and the HER2 pathway in breast cancer: effects of HER2 abundance. Transl Oncol 4:293–300

Farooqui M, Geng ZH, Stephenson EJ, Zaveri N, Yee D, Gupta K (2006) Naloxone acts as an antagonist of estrogen receptor activity in mcf-7 cells. Mol Cancer Ther 5:611–620. doi:5/3/611 [pii]10.1158/1535-7163.MCT-05-0016

Farooqui M, Li Y, Rogers T, Poonawala T, Griffin RJ, Song CW, Gupta K (2007) COX-2 inhibitor celecoxib prevents chronic morphine-induced promotion of angiogenesis, tumour growth, metastasis and mortality, without compromising analgesia. Br J Cancer 97:1523–1531

Finley MJ, Happel CM, Kaminsky DE, Rogers TJ (2008) Opioid and nociceptin receptors regulate cytokine and cytokine receptor expression. Cell Immunol 252:146–154

Fujioka N, Nguyen J, Chen C, Li Y, Pasrija T, Niehans G, Johnson KN, Gupta V, Kratzke RA, Gupta K (2011) Morphine-induced epidermal growth factor pathway activation in non-small cell lung cancer. Anesth Analg 113:1353–1364. doi:ANE.0b013e318232b35a [pii]10.1213/ANE.0b013e318232b35a

Gach K, Piestrzeniewicz M, Fichna J, Stefanska B, Szemraj J, Janecka A (2008) Opioid-induced regulation of mu-opioid receptor gene expression in the MCF-7 breast cancer cell line. Biochem Cell Biol 86:217–226

Gronemeyer H, Gustafsson JA, Laudet V (2004) Principles for modulation of the nuclear receptor superfamily. Nat Rev Drug Discov 3:950–964. doi:nrd1551 [pii]10.1038/nrd1551

Gupta K, Kshirsagar S, Chang L, Schwartz R, Law PY, Yee D, Hebbel RP (2002) Morphine stimulates angiogenesis by activating proangiogenic and survival-promoting signaling and promotes breast tumor growth. Cancer Res 62:4491–4498

Gupta M, Yunfang L, Gupta K (2007) Opioids as promoters and regulators of angiogenesis. In: Maragoudakis ME, Papadimitriou E (eds) Angiogenesis: basic science and clinical applications. Transworld Research Network, Kerala, pp 303–317

Gururaj AE, Rayala SK, Vadlamudi RK, Kumar R (2006) Novel mechanisms of resistance to endocrine therapy: genomic and nongenomic considerations. Clin Cancer Res 12:1001s–1007s

Hall JM, Couse JF, Korach KS (2001) The multifaceted mechanisms of estradiol and estrogen receptor signaling. J Biol Chem 276:36869–36872. doi:10.1074/jbc.R100029200R100029200 [pii]

Hall JM, McDonnell DP (1999) The estrogen receptor beta-isoform (erbeta) of the human estrogen receptor modulates eralpha transcriptional activity and is a key regulator of the cellular response to estrogens and antiestrogens. Endocrinology 140:5566–5578

Hammes SR, Levin ER (2007) Extranuclear steroid receptors: nature and actions. Endocr Rev 28:726–741. doi:er.2007-0022 [pii]10.1210/er.2007-0022

Hatzoglou A, Bakogeorgou E, Castanas E (1996a) The antiproliferative effect of opioid receptor agonists on the T47D human breast cancer cell line, is partially mediated through opioid receptors. Eur J Pharmacol 296:199–207. doi:0014-2999(95)00703-2 [pii]10.1016/0014-2999(95)00703-2

Hatzoglou A, Bakogeorgou E, Hatzoglou C, Martin PM, Castanas E (1996b) Antiproliferative and receptor binding properties of alpha- and beta-casomorphins in the T47D human breast cancer cell line. Eur J Pharmacol 310:217–223

Howe LR, Brown PH (2011) Targeting the her/egfr/erbb family to prevent breast cancer. Cancer Prev Res (Phila) 4:1149–1157. doi:4/8/1149 [pii]10.1158/1940-6207.CAPR-11-0334

Kajdaniuk D, Marek B, Swietochowska E, Ciesielska-Kopacz N, Buntner B (2000) Is positive correlation between cortisol and met-enkephalin concentration in blood of women with breast cancer a reaction to stress before chemotherapy administration? Pathophysiology 7:47–51

Kato S, Endoh H, Masuhiro Y, Kitamoto T, Uchiyama S, Sasaki H, Masushige S, Gotoh Y, Nishida E, Kawashima H, Metzger D, Chambon P (1995) Activation of the estrogen receptor through phosphorylation by mitogen-activated protein kinase. Science 270:1491–1494

Khan SA, Rogers MA, Obando JA, Tamsen A (1994) Estrogen receptor expression of benign breast epithelium and its association with breast cancer. Cancer Res 54:993–997

Koo KL, Tejwani GA, Abou-Issa H (1996) Relative efficacy of the opioid antagonist, naltrexone, on the initiation and promotion phases of rat mammary carcinogenesis. Anticancer Res 16:1893–1898

Korach KS, Emmen JM, Walker VR, Hewitt SC, Yates M, Hall JM, Swope DL, Harrell JC, Couse JF (2003) Update on animal models developed for analyses of estrogen receptor biological activity. J Steroid Biochem Mol Biol 86:387–391. doi:S0960076003003480 [pii]

Krege JH, Hodgin JB, Couse JF, Enmark E, Warner M, Mahler JF, Sar M, Korach KS, Gustafsson JA, Smithies O (1998) Generation and reproductive phenotypes of mice lacking estrogen receptor beta. Proc Natl Acad Sci U S A 95:15677–15682

Kugawa F, Arae K, Ueno A, Aoki M (1998) Buprenorphine hydrochloride induces apoptosis in ng108-15 nerve cells. Eur J Pharmacol 347:105–112. doi:S0014-2999(98)00080-6 [pii]

Lennon FE, Mirzapoiazova T, Mambetsariev B, Salgia R, Moss J, Singleton PA (2012) Overexpression of the mu-opioid receptor in human non-small cell lung cancer promotes Akt and mTOR activation, tumor growth, and metastasis. Anesthesiology. doi:10.1097/ALN.0b013e31824babe2

Lissoni P, Malugani F, Bordin V, Conti A, Maestroni G, Tancini G (2002) A new neuroimmunotherapeutic strategy of subcutaneous low-dose interleukin-2 plus the long-acting opioid antagonist naltrexone in metastatic cancer patients progressing on interleukin-2 alone. Neuro Endocrinol Lett 23:255–258

Lubahn DB, Moyer JS, Golding TS, Couse JF, Korach KS, Smithies O (1993) Alteration of reproductive function but not prenatal sexual development after insertional disruption of the mouse estrogen receptor gene. Proc Natl Acad Sci U S A 90:11162–11166

Lunzer MM, Yekkirala A, Hebbel RP, Portoghese PS (2007) Naloxone acts as a potent analgesic in transgenic mouse models of sickle cell anemia. Proc Natl Acad Sci U S A 104:6061–6065. doi:0700295104 [pii]10.1073/pnas.0700295104

Maneckjee R, Minna JD (1992) Nonconventional opioid binding sites mediate growth inhibitory effects of methadone on human lung cancer cells. Proc Natl Acad Sci U S A 89:1169–1173

Mangelsdorf DJ, Thummel C, Beato M, Herrlich P, Schutz G, Umesono K, Blumberg B, Kastner P, Mark M, Chambon P, Evans RM (1995) The nuclear receptor superfamily: the second decade. Cell 83:835–839. doi:0092-8674(95)90199-X [pii]

Massarweh S, Osborne CK, Creighton CJ, Qin L, Tsimelzon A, Huang S, Weiss H, Rimawi M, Schiff R (2008) Tamoxifen resistance in breast tumors is driven by growth factor receptor signaling with repression of classic estrogen receptor genomic function. Cancer Res 68:826–833. doi:68/3/826 [pii]10.1158/0008-5472.CAN-07-2707

Mathew B, Lennon FE, Siegler J, Mirzapoiazova T, Mambetsariev N, Sammani S, Gerhold LM, LaRiviere PJ, Chen CT, Garcia JG, Salgia R, Moss J, Singleton PA (2011) The novel role of the mu opioid receptor in lung cancer progression: a laboratory investigation. Anesth Analg 112:558–567. doi:ANE.0b013e31820568af [pii]10.1213/ANE.0b013e31820568af

McLaughlin PJ, Zagon IS (2012) The opioid growth factor-opioid growth factor receptor axis: Homeostatic regulator of cell proliferation and its implications for health and disease. Biochem Pharmacol 84:746–755

Moss J, Rosow CE (2008) Development of peripheral opioid antagonists' new insights into opioid effects. Mayo Clin Proc 83:1116–1130. doi:S0025-6196(11)60617-4 [pii]10.4065/83.10.1116

Nilsson S, Koehler KF, Gustafsson JA (2011) Development of subtype-selective oestrogen receptor-based therapeutics. Nat Rev Drug Discov 10:778–792. doi:nrd3551 [pii]10.1038/nrd3551

Panagiotou S, Hatzoglou A, Calvo F, Martin PM, Castanas E (1998) Modulation of the estrogen-regulated proteins cathepsin D and pS2 by opioid agonists in hormone-sensitive breast cancer cell lines (MCF7 and T47D): evidence for an interaction between the two systems. J Cell Biochem 71:416–428. doi:10.1002/(SICI)1097-4644(19981201)71:3<416::AID-JCB10>3.0.CO;2-Y [pii]

Power I (2011) An update on analgesics. Br J Anaesth 107:19–24. doi:aer126 [pii]10.1093/bja/aer126

Ring A, Dowsett M (2004) Mechanisms of tamoxifen resistance. Endocr Relat Cancer 11:643–658

Sinchak K, Micevych PE (2001) Progesterone blockade of estrogen activation of mu-opioid receptors regulates reproductive behavior. J Neurosci 21:5723–5729. doi:21/15/5723 [pii]

Singleton PA, Lingen MW, Fekete MJ, Garcia JG, Moss J (2006) Methylnaltrexone inhibits opiate and VEGF-induced angiogenesis: role of receptor transactivation. Microvasc Res 72:3–11. doi:S0026-2862(06)00043-4 [pii]10.1016/j.mvr.2006.04.004

Singleton PA, Garcia JG, Moss J (2008) Synergistic effects of methylnaltrexone with 5-fluorouracil and bevacizumab on inhibition of vascular endothelial growth factor-induced angiogenesis. Mol Cancer Ther 7:1669–1679

Singleton PA, Mambetsariev N, Lennon FE, Mathew B, Siegler JH, Moreno-Vinasco L, Salgia R, Moss J, Garcia JG (2010) Methylnaltrexone potentiates the anti-angiogenic effects of mTOR inhibitors. J Angiogenes Res 2:5. doi:2040-2384-2-5 [pii]10.1186/2040-2384-2-5

Stephenson EJ, Gupta K (2006) Existence and modus operandi of opioid receptors in endothelium. In: Aird W (ed) The endothelium: a comprehensive reference. Cambridge University Press, Cambridge, MA, pp 451–460

Tegeder I, Grosch S, Schmidtko A, Haussler A, Schmidt H, Niederberger E, Scholich K, Geisslinger G (2003) G protein-independent g1 cell cycle block and apoptosis with morphine in adenocarcinoma cells: involvement of p53 phosphorylation. Cancer Res 63:1846–1852

Tsunashima K (1982) Anticancer effect of naloxone. Proc Jpn Cancer Assoc 425

Vogel VG, Costantino JP, Wickerham DL, Cronin WM, Cecchini RS, Atkins JN, Bevers TB, Fehrenbacher L, Pajon ER, Wade JL 3rd, Robidoux A, Margolese RG, James J, Runowicz CD, Ganz PA, Reis SE, McCaskill-Stevens W, Ford LG, Jordan VC, Wolmark N (2010) Update of the national surgical adjuvant breast and bowel project study of tamoxifen and raloxifene (STAR) P-2 trial: preventing breast cancer. Cancer Prev Res (Phila) 3:696–706. doi:1940-6207.CAPR-10-0076 [pii]10.1158/1940-6207.CAPR-10-0076

Wu Q, Chambliss K, Umetani M, Mineo C, Shaul PW (2011) Non-nuclear estrogen receptor signaling in the endothelium. J Biol Chem 286:14737–14743. doi:R110.191791 [pii]10.1074/jbc.R110.191791

Zagon IS, McLaughlin PJ (1983a) Naltrexone modulates tumor response in mice with neuroblastoma. Science 221:671–673

Zagon IS, McLaughlin PJ (1983b) Opioid antagonists inhibit the growth of metastatic murine neuroblastoma. Cancer Lett 21:89–94

Zagon IS, McLaughlin PJ (1987) Modulation of murine neuroblastoma in nude mice by opioid antagonists. J Natl Cancer Inst 78:141–147

Zagon IS, Donahue RN, McLaughlin PJ (2009) Opioid growth factor-opioid growth factor receptor axis is a physiological determinant of cell proliferation in diverse human cancers. Am J Physiol Regul Integr Comp Physiol 297:R1154–R1161

# Chapter 3
# Morphine and Immunosuppression in the Context of Tumor Growth and Metastasis

**Lisa Koodie and Sabita Roy**

**Abstract** Morphine has been recognized as a highly potent analgesic agent used in cancer and non-cancer (neuropathic, surgical) pain management. Cancer patients may be prescribed morphine at different stages of the disease, during neoplastic growth and progression, during surgical resection and even in end stage palliative care. Morphine has been shown to suppress immune cell activation, functionality and cytokine secretion. While the initial infiltration of immune cells during tumor growth can be beneficial in destroying stressed tumor cells, prolonged accumulation results in a dampened immune response, enhanced angiogenesis, tumor growth and thus metastasis. The aim of this chapter is summarize the immunosuppressive effects of morphine as it relates to metastasis. We describe the effects of morphine as it pertains to tumor cell proliferation and growth, immune cell contribution to angiogenesis and extracellular matrix remodeling within the tumor microenvironment.

**Keywords** Immunosuppression • Macrophages • Mast cells • Morphine • Myeloid suppressor cells • Natural killer cells • Neutrophils • T cells

---

L. Koodie
Department of Dentistry, Division of Basic Translational Research, University of Minnesota, Mayo Mail Code 195, 420 Delaware Street SE, Minneapolis, MN 55455, USA

S. Roy (✉)
Department of Pharmacology and Department of Surgery, Division of Basic Translational Research, University of Minnesota, Mayo Mail Code 195, 420 Delaware Street SE, Minneapolis, MN 55455, USA
e-mail: royxx002@umn.edu

M.-O. Parat (ed.), *Morphine and Metastasis*, DOI 10.1007/978-94-007-5678-6_3, 

## Abbreviations

| | |
|---|---|
| CTL | cytolytic T lymphocyte |
| ELISA | enzyme-linked immuno-sorbent assay |
| fMLP | formyl-methionyl-leucyl-phenylalanine |
| HSV-1 | herpes simplex virus type 1 |
| HPA | hypothalamic pituitary axis |
| HIF1α | hypoxia inducible transcription factor |
| IgG | immunoglobulin-G |
| iNOS | inducible nitric oxide synthase |
| IL | interleukin |
| KC/CXCL1 | keratinocyte-derived cytokine |
| LPS | lipopolysaccharide |
| MIP | macrophage inflammatory protein |
| MMP | matrix metalloprotease |
| MAPK | mitogen activated protein kinase |
| MOR | mu-opioid receptor |
| MDSC | myeloid derived suppressor cells |
| MSC | myeloid suppressor cells |
| NOP | non classical-nociceptin/orphanin FQ receptor |
| NF-κB | nuclear factor kappa B |
| PMA | phorbol 12-myristate 13-acetate |
| RANTES | regulated upon activation normal T cell expressed |
| SCF | stem cell factor |
| SDF-1 | stromal derived factor-1 |
| Th1 | T cell helper 1 |
| Th2 | T cell helper 2 |
| TGF-β | transforming growth factor beta |
| TNF-α | tumor necrosis factor alpha |
| VCAM-1 | vascular cell adhesion molecule-1 |
| VEGF | vascular endothelial growth factor |

## 3.1 Introduction

The immunosuppressive effects of morphine result from both direct and indirect actions. Morphine can exert direct effects on immune cells expressing the opioid receptors. Morphine can also act indirectly through the central nervous system, and by hypothalamic pituitary axis (HPA) activation. To date, morphine has been recognized as a highly potent analgesic agent used in cancer and non-cancer (neuropathic, surgical) pain management. Cancer patients may be prescribed morphine at different stages of the disease, during neoplastic growth and progression, during surgical resection and even in end stage palliative care. Importantly, not all opioids exert the same level of immunosuppression. For example the potent opioid fentanyl exhibits greater immunosuppression than buprenorphine – a partial agonist that has less immunosuppressive effects. Similarly, hydromorphone and oxycodone appear to have no effect on immunosuppression (Pergolizzi et al. 2009; Güttler and Sabatowski 2008). On the other hand, other opiate agonists like Tramadol have been shown to be immuno-stimulatory (Shirzad et al. 2009). The aim of this chapter is to summarize the immunosuppressive effects of morphine as they relate to tumor growth and metastasis.

## 3.2 Major Contributors of Tumor Cell Metastasis

There are over 100 types of different cancers, each named for their cellular origin but characterized similarly – as cells that grow out of control. Although this uncontrollable proliferation is balanced by cell death initially during the early stages of cancer development, in some cases that balance is tipped to cell proliferation and a mass of cells is formed, commonly referred to as a solid tumor. Tumors are further sub-divided into benign or malignant. Benign tumors are characterized as cells with limited growth potential and usually stay at the site of origin. In the case of malignant tumors, tumor cells move from the original site through the blood and lymph systems and invade otherwise healthy organs. When the tumor successfully spreads and grows, it is said to have metastasized, or undergone metastasis. Tumor cell-secreted chemokines attract bone marrow, myeloid-derived leukocytes that eventually contribute to angiogenesis, forming vessels that are the primary route of tumor cell metastasis.

The immune system has a dual role in tumor growth. Rudolf Virchow was the first scientist to make the observation that infiltrating leukocytes were abundant in cancer tissues. During the early stages of tumor growth, immune cells are capable of recognizing stressed tumor cells and promote an effective immune response leading to tumor cell death. In solid tumors that escape this immune surveillance and grow beyond 1–2 $mm^3$, the formation of new blood vessels, termed angiogenesis, occurs as a result of hypoxia-induced tumor cell growth factor secretion (Ye et al. 2010; Lewis and Murdoch 2005).

Rapid cancer cell proliferation ultimately determines the extent in which the tumor grows. Any reduction in cell growth would therefore decrease the rate of solid tumor formation. If the tumor does not grow beyond the size necessary to elicit blood vessel formation, then metastasis would be unlikely. In the next section we review the current literature on the effects of morphine on cancer cell proliferation and tumor growth.

## 3.3 Effects of Morphine on Cancer Cell Proliferation and Tumor Growth

The effects of morphine on tumor cell proliferation in vitro vary depending on the cell type and concentration of morphine tested. Morphine (10 μM) inhibited the proliferation of breast cancer cells MCF-7 and MDA-MB231 and increased cell death (>500 μM) in vitro. Morphine also reduced tumor growth when MCF-7 and MDA-MB231 were injected subcutaneously in nude mice but had no effect on HT-29, a human colon adenocarcinoma grade II cell line (Tegeder et al. 2003). Although MCF-7 and MDA-MB231 cells responded to morphine by classical opioid receptors signaling cascade activation, morphine-induced inhibition of tumor cell proliferation and tumor growth were found to be independent of this pathway, since they were not reversed in the presence of naloxone or pertussis toxin. Morphine inhibition of tumor cell proliferation and growth in MCF-7 and MDA-MB231 was proposed to be due to an increase in tumor suppressor protein p53 activation that increased the death proteins p21, Bax, and the death receptor Fas. Furthermore, blockade of Fas or inhibition of caspase 8 partially reduced the morphine-induced apoptosis of MCF-7 and MDA-MB231 cells (Tegeder et al. 2003). In contrast, HT-29 cells were found to express a dominant negative p53 and were incapable of increased GTPase activity after morphine treatment.

In another study, when MDA-MB-231 (oestrogen positive) and MCF7 (oestrogen negative) breast cancer cells were incubated with morphine at 10–100 ng/ml, an increase in cell proliferation over control was observed (Ecimovic et al. 2011). In this study the authors assessed the expression of NET1 in the presence of morphine. The gene product of NET1 has a key role in actin reorganization and was found to be over-expressed in breast and gastric adenocarcinoma cells where it may contribute to increased migration and invasion. These studies suggest that morphine increases NET1 gene expression, and breast cancer cell migration (using fetal bovine serum as the chemoattractant) in an in vitro chemotaxis assay. Silencing RNA to NET1 abolished the morphine-induced increase in cell migration. Interestingly, when the investigators used real time PCR to evaluate opioid receptor expression, they found that the non-classical nociceptin/orphanin FQ (NOP) receptor was expressed in MCF-7 cells and that the delta opioid receptor was expressed in MDA-MB-231 cells. However, the other classical opioid receptors, namely mu- or kappa-opioid receptors, were absent. Of note, these investigators did not measure the protein levels of NET1, and the lack of mu-opioid receptors makes it difficult to fully extrapolate these findings to a clinical setting. In vitro studies conducted by Hatsukari and colleagues revealed that morphine (10 nM) within clinically relevant concentrations (0.9–3.4 μM) induced early apoptotic markers (such as Annexin V) and decreased cell viability in HL-60 (human promyelocytic leukemia cells), and A549 (human lung adenocarcinoma epithelial cell line) while causing necrosis in MCF-7 cells. Additionally, these effects were naloxone-reversible (Hatsukari et al. 2007).

Taken together these studies suggest that morphine may produce direct effects on tumor cells within the tumor microenvironment. Apoptotic and or necrotic tumor cells would eventually attract inflammatory leukocytes to remove dead and dying tumor cells. The recruited inflammatory cells, while beneficial in removing the dead tumor cells, also receive cues from hypoxic tumor cells and contribute to angiogenesis within the developing solid tumor.

## 3.4 Immune Cells That Contribute to Tumor Growth and Metastasis

Morphine modulates both functionality and intracellular signaling in cells of the innate and acquired immune systems. Morphine is capable of inhibiting many innate and adaptive immune cell functions in vitro. Numerous studies have identified important intracellular signaling pathways involved in morphine-induced immunosuppression (reviewed in Roy et al. 2011).

### *3.4.1 Myeloid Suppressor Cells*

Myeloid-derived suppressor cells or myeloid suppressor cells (MDSC, MSCs) play a key role in cancer invasion and metastasis through the secretion of pro-angiogenic factors (vascular endothelial growth factor, VEGF), enzymes such as matrix metalloproteases (MMPs), and chemokines. In hypoxic regions of solid tumors, expression by tumor cells of hypoxia-inducible factor (HIF)1$\alpha$ is induced. HIF-1$\alpha$ is a hypoxia-induced transcription factor whose protein stability and gene regulation mediate tumor cell secretion of stromal derived factor-1 (SDF-1), stem cell factor (SCF), CXCL5 and CCL2. MSCs have been found in human head and neck cancer, renal cell carcinoma, non-small-cell lung cancer, colon and breast cancers, colorectal, malignant melanoma, hepato-cellular carcinoma, pancreatic cancer, Hodgkin lymphoma, non-Hodgkin lymphoma, and even multiple myeloma (Ye et al. 2010; Tadmor et al. 2011). MSC are a heterogeneous population of monocytes and granulocytes that include immature macrophages, dendritic cells, neutrophils and other myeloid cells at multiple stages of differentiation (Ye et al. 2010). Inflammatory monocytes and immature neutrophils have been shown to suppress T cell responses (Movahedi et al. 2008). The knock down of SCF expression in mice with subcutaneous tumor cells treated with siRNA for SCF resulted in a reduction in MSC expansion and restoration of tumor infiltrating T cell proliferative ability (Pan et al. 2008).

Currently no studies exist on the effect of morphine on MSC formation, migration and establishment within the tumor site.

### *3.4.2 Macrophages*

The tumor-associated macrophages and M2 macrophages secrete cytokines (interleukin (IL)-10) and growth factors (transforming growth factor beta) and display immunosuppressive behaviors. In contrast to M2, the M1 macrophages are immuno-stimulatory, and secrete factors such as NO (from inducible nitric oxide synthase (iNOS)), (IL)-12 and tumor necrosis factor that contributes to tumor cell death (Vasievich and Huang 2011; Tadmor et al. 2011). M2 macrophages secrete proangiogenic factors (such as vascular endothelial growth factor – VEGF) that promote further recruitment of monocytes which differentiate within the tumor microenvironment and participate in angiogenesis (Murdoch et al. 2008). Monocyte-derived macrophages secrete additional growth factors once recruited to the tumor site, but the initial expression of such factors within the tumor microenvironment is predominantly from hypoxic tumor cells and/or endothelial cells.

Acute morphine treatment of human macrophages was shown to result in a transient inhibition in macrophage cell migration and increased iNOS production (Stefano et al. 2001). Studies in mice show that morphine but not corticosterone activates macrophage nitric oxide production (Wang et al. 2002). Morphine withdrawal reduces plaque-forming cell response of mouse spleen macrophages to sheep red blood cells in vitro (Rahim et al. 2005). Interestingly, in RAW 264 cells, a mouse leukemic monocyte macrophage cell line, transfected with the human VEGF promoter linked to a firefly luciferase, inflammatory mediators and hypoxia increased luciferase expression, suggesting VEGF promoter activation in response to such stimuli. However, morphine pretreatment significantly reduced promoter activation upon inflammatory mediator or hypoxia stimulation (Martin et al. 2010). This result was confirmed by assessing VEGF protein secretion. Enzyme-linked immunosorbent assay (ELISA) confirmed that RAW264 cells secreted VEGF in response to inflammatory mediators, and this was decreased with morphine pretreatment. Although whether these effects of morphine were through mu opioid receptor (MOR) was not established or confirmed, hypoxia-induced HIF1α protein localization to the nucleus (which mediates VEGF transcription and thus secretion) was disrupted after morphine pretreatment (Martin et al. 2010). These results provide a molecular basis for inhibition by morphine of hypoxia-induced VEGF expression in macrophages.

Morphine was found to decrease the recruitment of monocytes (Ly6C, Tie2), neutrophils (Ly6G, Gr1) and macrophages (F4/80) into inert PVA sponges implanted subcutaneously into mice and containing inflammatory or tumor cell-derived chemoattractants (Martin et al. 2010, Koodie L unpublished observations). The effect of morphine on peripheral macrophage and brain-associated microglia (brain macrophages) migration is another important question to address, related to metastasis. Potentially, a reduction in macrophage-monocyte migration into the tumor would lead to reduced angiogenesis and thus decreased metastasis. Morphine has been shown to reduce macrophage and microglial migration towards chemokines in vitro. The production of the chemokine Regulated upon activation, normal T cell expressed and secreted (RANTES) by primary cultures of human microglial cells in response to inflammatory mediators (lipopolysaccharide (LPS), IL-1β) was blunted by morphine treatment, as was chemotaxis of microglial cells towards RANTES. This effect was reversed with naloxone and beta-funaltrexamine, indicating involvement of mu-opioid receptors (Hu et al. 2000). In a urinary tract infection model, morphine treatment increased the apoptosis of murine bone marrow cells and inhibited macrophage migration when tested in an *in vitro* chemotaxis assay and in vivo within the peritoneal cavity (Malik et al. 2002).

The ability of undifferentiated circulating monocytes to differentiate into macrophages once within the tumor microenvironment may also represent a major aspect in angiogenesis. Phorbol 12-myristate 13-acetate (PMA) can induce the differentiation of THP-1 monocytes into macrophages and increase their adhesion to substrates and migration capacity in vitro (Hatsukari et al. 2006). Morphine can prevent this monocyte-macrophage differentiation, as in the presence of morphine PMA stimulation of THP-1 differentiation, adhesion, and migration is blunted (Hatsukari et al. 2006).

Taken together, acute and chronic morphine treatment and even withdrawal can exert suppressive effects on macrophage function and growth factor expression. Although more direct studies are necessary, morphine may hinder macrophage contribution to angiogenesis, a primary route for tumor metastasis, and thus possibly contribute to a net reduction in metastasis.

### *3.4.3 Neutrophils*

Neutrophil-secreted cytokines and chemokines promote inflammatory cell recruitment and activation. Neutrophil products such as VEGF, reactive oxygen species and MMPs affect many aspects of tumor cell growth, angiogenesis and metastasis (reviewed in Gregory and Houghton 2011). Literature on the direct effects of morphine on neutrophils in the context of tumor growth and metastasis is limited. Studies from independent investigators utilizing different models of infection, showed that morphine increased bacterial dissemination and reduced bacterial clearance in mice, when compared to saline as a result of poor neutrophil recruitment (Wang et al. 2005; Breslow et al. 2011). In response to intranasal *Streptococcus pneumoniae*, morphine significantly decreased the tumor necrosis factor alpha (TNF-α), interleukin-1, interleukin-6, macrophage inflammatory protein (MIP)-2, and keratinocyte-derived cytokines (KC/CXCL1) in bronchoalveolar lavage fluids and lung tissue (Wang et al. 2005). In response to intraperitoneal *Acinetobacter baumannii*, morphine decreased expression of neutrophil-inducing molecules, interleukin-17A and KC/CXCL1, potentiating such infection (Breslow et al. 2011).

Morphine is administered before, during and after tumor resection. In an incisional model in mice, acute morphine administration reduced neutrophil infiltration into the incision site and lowered the amounts of interleukin-1 beta, interleukin-6, tumor necrosis factor alpha, granulocyte colony stimulating factor and keratinocyte-derived cytokine (Clark et al. 2007). Similarly, morphine decreased carrageenan-induced hindpaw swelling and myeloperoxidase (expressed predominantly in neutrophil-monocytes) in Fischer 344 and Lewis rats, but did not significantly alter circulating cytokines (Fecho et al. 2007). In vitro models investigating the direct effects of morphine on neutrophil chemotaxis to interleukin-8 (IL-8) show that morphine inhibits IL-8 induced chemotaxis of human neonatal neutrophils as a result of downregulation of IL-8 receptor expression, but this effect is not seen with human adult neutrophils (Yossuck et al. 2008). Similar observations were made of morphine affecting monkey neutrophil chemotaxis towards IL-8 and monkey monocyte chemotaxis to RANTES as the chemoattractant (Miyagi et al. 2000; Choi et al. 1999).

The activation of the transcription factor nuclear factor kappa B (NF-κB) has been investigated as one mechanism of morphine-induced immunosuppression in neutrophils and monocytes. NF-κB is essential in the LPS-induced inflammatory response and leukocyte activation. Morphine suppresses LPS-induced NF-κB activation in human monocytes and neutrophils and this effect is reversed in the presence of naloxone. The effect of morphine on nuclear binding of NF-κB is similar to that observed with nitric oxide donors, and NOS inhibitors have shown to be effective in abolishing morphine's inhibitory effects on NF-κB activation (Welters et al. 2000a). Morphine but not fentanyl inhibited complement and Fc-γ receptor expression in human neutrophils (Welters et al. 2000b).

Neutrophils could potentially participate in tumor growth through de-granulation and thus death of tumor cells but in an environment where stressed or hypoxic cells accumulate, facilitate tumor growth, angiogenesis and metastasis. Inhibitory effects of morphine on neutrophil function and migration could potentially reduce angiogenesis and thus metastasis.

### *3.4.4 T Cells*

Lymphocytes also infiltrate solid tumors. Tumor-infiltrating T cell contribution to tumor growth varies depending on the subset in query, tumor type, CD4+:CD8+ ratios and location within the tumor (near epithelium versus within cancer stroma). Infiltration of CD8+ T cells into tumors or at metastatic sites is generally associated with positive outcomes, in contrast to CD4+ T cells that are associated with poor survival (Talmadge 2011). T cells have been found in pancreatic ductal adenocarcinoma, renal clear cell carcinoma, hepatocarcinoma, cutaneous melanoma, non-small lung carcinoma, and ovarian and colorectal carcinomas. Tumor-derived chemokines prevent immature MSCs from activating T cells. Within the tumor, MSCs increase their secretion of IL-10, TGF-β, and inducible nitric oxide synthase that arrest T-cell cycling and proliferation (Talmadge 2011). T cells within tumors respond poorly to antigens and this reduces their ability to kill tumor cells.

T cells do express the mu-opioid receptor which is up-regulated by chronic morphine treatment and CD3/28 activation (Campana et al. 2010; Börner et al. 2008). Through action on the MOR, morphine suppresses the CD3/CD28 induction of IL-2 gene expression and protein secretion via effects on calcium and mitogen-activated protein kinase (MAPK) activation (Liu et al. 2006; Wang et al. 2007; Börner et al. 2008, 2009). Antibody activation of CD3/CD28 in spleen-derived T lymphocytes increases IL-4 promoter activity and increases IL-4 protein secretion in vitro. Chronic morphine treatment synergistically increased IL-4 promoter activity and protein secretion upon antibody-induced CD3/CD28 activation, resulting in preferential enhancement of T helper (Th)2 cell differentiation (Roy et al. 2005; Greeneltch et al. 2005; Azarang et al. 2007) and Th1 killing in a Fas/FasL dependent mechanism (Greeneltch et al. 2005).

IL-2 is a cytokine expressed by activated CD4+ T cells. IL-2 promotes naïve T cell proliferation and expansion of CD8+ T cells, induces the differentiation of regulatory T cells and promotes the development of cytotoxic T lymphocytes. Depending on the cytokine milieu, IL-2 can promote Th-1 differentiation but inhibit Th-17 differentiation. Cells expressing the IL-2 receptor family of proteins include T, B, natural killer (NK) cells and neutrophils, and they respond to IL-2 signaling (Liao et al. 2011). IL-4 was first identified as a T cell-secreted factor capable of stimulating B-cell proliferation and immunoglobulin-G (IgG) class switching. IL-4 has both anti and pro-tumorigenic activites. The tumor-promoting effects of IL-4 include promotion of tumor-associated macrophage activity, pro-angiogenesis (via the ability to up-regulate soluble vascular cell adhesion molecule-1 (VCAM-1)), slowing of the progression of T cell-mediated immunity against tumor cells, reduction of tumor cell apoptosis in some tumors and enhanced cell proliferation. Anti-tumor effects of IL-4 occur through the recruitment and activation of innate immune cells (neutrophils, eosinophils and dendritic cells), enhancement of CD8+ T cells-anti tumor immunity, induction of apoptosis in tumor cells, as well inhibition of angiogenesis through direct effects on endothelial cells or indirect effects on tumor stromal fibroblasts (Wang and Joyce 2010).

In patients undergoing gastric cancer surgery, morphine was given intravenously for pain relief and compared to tramadol only or tramadol with lornoxicam. Analysis of lymphocyte subsets in peripheral blood from patients showed no difference at baseline amongst patients receiving different medications. The surgery itself decreased total lymphocytes in all patient groups. However, starting 90 min and up to 48 h post-surgery, morphine-receiving patients had a significant decrease of T lymphocytes (CD3+; CD3+/CD4+; ratio CD3+/CD4:CD3/CD8+) from baseline numbers, with a slight but insignificant increase in CD3/CD8+ lymphocytes. The natural killer cells and activated lymphocytes were also lower in patients receiving morphine, when compared to tramadol (Wang et al. 2006). Morphine suppresses the generation of human cytotoxic T lymphocytes but enhances cytolytic activity against Human T-lymphotropic virus Type I (HTLV-I)-induced T-cell leukemia cells in vitro (Fugetta et al. 2005). In a model of herpes simplex virus type 1 (HSV-1) infection, acute morphine administration was found to significantly reduce cytolytic T lymphocyte activity, lymphocyte proliferation, and IFN-gamma production (Mojadadi et al. 2009). A reduction in cytolytic activity can potentially increase tumor growth and thus metastasis. In vitro assays using a T-cell hybridoma, mouse splenocytes, and freshly isolated human peripheral blood lymphocytes, showed that morphine, through the opiate receptors (naloxone reversible), dramatically increases the expression of Fas and thus apoptosis of T cells which contributes to its immunosuppressive effects (Yin et al. 1999). The Fas death Receptor and Fas Ligand have been implicated in morphine-induced immunosuppression (Greeneltch et al. 2005; Yin et al. 2006). In contrast, studies using freshly isolated human peripheral blood-derived lymphocytes showed that 48 h in vitro morphine treatment was not sufficient to induce Fas, Bcl-2 or caspase-3 activity (Ohara et al. 2005).

The ability of morphine to tip the balance towards a shift in Th2 responses, and a decrease in Th1 responses would suggest a decrease in effective tumor cell killing but possibly an increased B-cell antibody response. Lymphocyte levels are modulated with surgery, and morphine given for pain management can reduce circulating

CD4+T cells with little effect on CD8+ T cells. Patients given morphine for pain management may be exposed to high concentrations and may experience withdrawal, or cycle between high and low plasma concentrations. The exact mechanisms underlying morphine-induced immunosuppression is still not well understood and may vary between immune cell type and with the environment. Studies from *in vivo* models suggest that chronic morphine treatment results in thymic and spleen atrophy (Sedqi, et al. 1995; Freier and Fuchs 1993). The immunosuppressive effects induced by an acute administration of morphine differ from chronic effects and withdrawal effects. The impact of long-term morphine treatment, withdrawal and morphine tolerance on cytotoxic CD8+ lymphocytes function and their relationship to tumor progression, remains to be investigated.

### *3.4.5 Natural Killer Cells*

In several mouse models, NK cells have demonstrated their ability to suppress tumor growth and metastasis by exerting direct cytotoxic effects and enhancing tumor cell apoptosis, secretion of immune-stimulatory cytokines that boosts the adaptive immune response, and inhibition of tumor cell proliferation and angiogenesis (reviewed in Levy et al. 2011). In human studies, low NK cell activity is often associated with increased metastasis (Franchi et al. 2007). In addition to CD4+/CD8+ T cells, myeloid suppressor cells interact with natural killer cells. NK cells have been shown to participate in tumor suppression through the secretion of IL-13. IL-13 contributes to MSC suppression of T-regulatory cell formation. Another mechanism by which MSCs alter NK activity is through the inhibition of macrophage IL-12 and TGFβ production. Adoptive cell transfer or antibody-stimulation of NK cells has been an attractive strategy to suppress cancer progression (Levy et al. 2011).

Patients given high dose fentanyl after esophageal cancer surgery showed a reduction in NK cell number assessed in peripheral blood post-surgery when compared to pre-surgery. High dose fentanyl (20 μg/ml) produced a more suppressive effect than lower doses (5–10 μg/ml) at 24–48 h post surgery (Li et al. 2003). In rodents, surgical stress itself has been closely associated with decreased NK activity and enhancement of tumor cell metastasis. In a mouse model of surgical stress, morphine and fentanyl, when compared to buprenorphine, stimulated the hypothalamic pituitary adrenal (HPA) axis, decreased NK cell activity and had no effect on stress-induced tumor metastasis. Unlike morphine and fentanyl, buprenorphine reversed the surgical stress-induced increase in tumor metastasis (Franchi et al. 2007). Similar results were seen when morphine was administered in rat mesencephalon periaqueductal gray. Morphine-treated mice displayed suppressed splenic NK cell cytotoxic activity compared to saline-injected mice (Liang-Suo et al. 2002).

Conflicting results from studies testing the effects of morphine on MADB106 adenocarcinoma cell metastasis to lung during surgical stress make it difficult to assess the potential effect of morphine on NK cell's ability to control tumor cell metastasis. In one study, morphine significantly decreased NK cell cytotoxicity in normal rats and did not prevent surgery-induced immunosuppression as seen with tramadol (Gaspani et al. 2002). In another study, laparotomy conducted under halothane anesthesia alone increased lung tumor retention up to 17-fold and this was reduced when combined with bupivacaine and morphine. Systemic morphine combined with halothane anesthesia reduced the effects of surgery, but to a lesser extent than halothane anesthesia with bupivacaine and morphine (Bar-Yosef et al. 2001). In a macaque model, significant decreases in the absolute number and percentage of NK cells have been observed during morphine dependence (chronic treatment over months). Interestingly, precipitated withdrawal or morphine abstinence (24 h) significantly increased the percentage of NK cells when compared to morphine dependence (Weed et al. 2006).

Increased functionality and recruitment of NK cells to the developing tumor may help control tumor cell proliferation and angiogenesis. Morphine has various effects on the number of NK cells circulating post surgery and that can potentially reduce immune surveillance and increase the chances of metastasis. Most of what we know about morphine effects on NK cells comes from non-human models and more studies are necessary to further understand the effects of morphine on NK cell functionality.

### *3.4.6 Mast Cells*

The exact contribution of mast cells to cancer metastasis is still not completely understood. Mast cells have been found to accumulate at the periphery of solid tumors such as oral squamous cell carcinoma (Kalra et al. 2011), colon cancer (Xia et al. 2011), cutaneous melanoma (Maltby et al. 2011), cervical carcinoma (Diaconu et al. 2011), pancreatic ductal adenocarcinoma (Cai et al. 2011), endometrioid adenocarcinoma of endometrium (Pansrikaew et al. 2010), breast cancer (Xiang et al. 2010) and gastric carcinoma (Ribatti et al. 2010). While the exact functional role of mast cells at the tumor periphery is still debated, it may well be dependent on the origin of the cancer cells and chemokine environment. Mast cells are cytotoxic to tumor cells, but also contain histamine, heparin, proteases, and MMPs that together promote extracellular matrix remodeling and neovascularisation. Physiologically, the proteolytic remodeling functions of mast cell-derived MMPs are necessary in developmental tissue morphogenesis, tissue repair, and angiogenesis. However, excessive release of MMPs leads to eventual tissue destruction creating an environment appropriate for tumor cell metastasis.

In mice with high mast cell numbers, acute morphine increases mast cell proliferation and recruitment to the peritoneal cavity in response to zymosan *in vivo* (Wypasek et al. 2011). Morphine also induces histamine degranulation by mast cells derived from CBA mice but not SWISS mice (Stankiewicz et al. 2004). In studies using LPS as the inflammatory stimuli, morphine decreased mast cell LPS-induced TNFα but not CCL2 secretion (Madera-Salcedo et al. 2011). Mast cell secretion of TNFα affects endothelial cell signaling, allowing for effective transmigration of more leukocytes from the circulation into tissues. Morphine and codeine induce mast cell degranulation independent of mu-opioid receptor signaling. *In vitro* studies comparing the two opiates codeine and meperidine showed that codeine, but not meperidine, activated human mast cell (LAD2 cell line, CD34+ cells) degranulation within 30 min of treatment. At 3 and 8 h, unlike meperidine, codeine was also able to activate human-derived mast cell release of monocyte chemoattractant protein-1/CCL2, RANTES/CCL5 and interleukin-8/CXCL-8 but not inducible protein-10 (Sheen et al. 2007). In contrast, using the human mast cell line HMC-1, clinically relevant concentrations of morphine (0.018–0.45 μg/ml) did not significantly increase histamine release. Interestingly, a higher concentration of morphine (668 μg/ml) was required to induce histamine release (Gordon et al. 2004). Histamine-containing mast cells degranulate in response to formyl-Methionyl-Leucyl-Phenylalanine (fMLP). In an *in vivo* model using the intact and isolated distal ileal mucosa of Sprague–Dawley rats, exposure to fMLP led to an increase in the permeability of dextran beads. Morphine treatment, similar to mast cell degranulation inhibitors (doxantrazole) or to mast cell deficient mice, reduced this fMLP-induced permeability (Harari et al. 2006). Morphine-induced mast cell degranulation has been reported for human cells (Miller et al. 1997). In swine however, an *in vivo* model assessing the inflammatory response after the intradermal inoculation of the compound 48/80, showed that morphine-tolerant swine had a significantly decreased amount of 48/80-induced infiltrating mast cells (Risdahl et al. 1995).

Mast cells can be cytotoxic to tumor cells, but also promote extracellular matrix remodeling and neovascularisation. Morphine may stimulate human mast cell line degranulation, inhibit TNFα secretion reduce FMLP induced mucosal permeability as well as mast cell recruitment to sites of inflammation *in vivo*. However more studies are required to understand the effects of morphine on mast cells.

## 3.5 Concluding Remarks

The development of blood vessels within solid tumors contributes to the metastatic process. Once vessels are formed and even though they are of poor integrity, agents that modulate vascular permeability can be expected to modulate tumor cell dissemination and thus metastasis. Morphine can act on other cells in the tumor system, altering protein expression of numerous growth factors and chemokines that cross-talk to the immune system. Here we reviewed the immunosuppressive effects of morphine as they pertain to metastasis (Fig. 3.1). Modulating the immune cell contribution to tumor cell growth, development and maintenance of angiogenesis as well as extracellular matrix remodeling within the tumor microenvironment may provide attractive therapeutic strategies to control tumor cell metastasis. Morphine has been shown to have direct effects on immune cell chemotactic migration, inflammatory stimuli cytokine secretion and functionality. Over-activation and continual recruitment of tumor infiltrating leukocytes into solid tumors can be potentially modulated with morphine treatment.

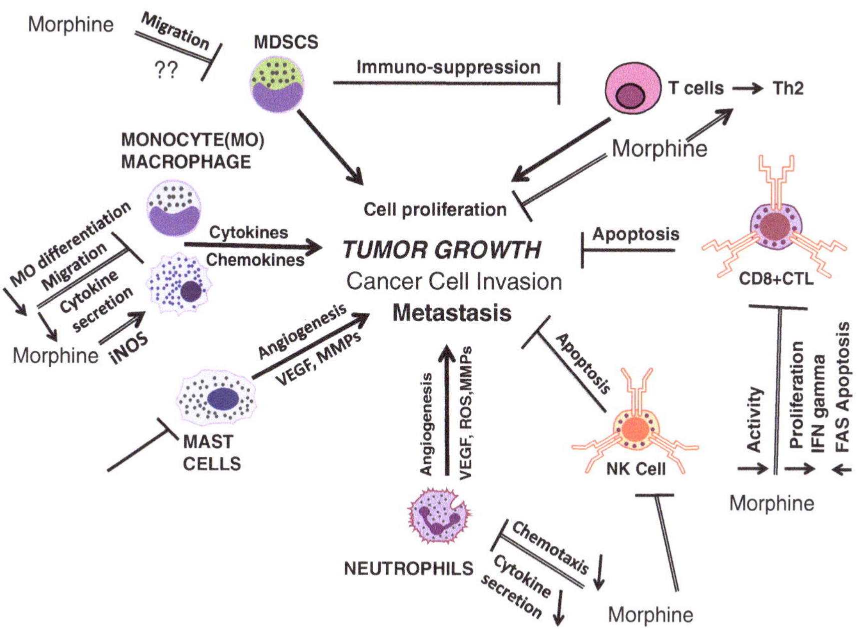


**Fig. 3.1** Schematic showing the effects of morphine on aspects of metastasis

# References

Azarang A, Mahmoodi M, Rajabalian S, Shekari MA, Nosratabadi J, Rezaei N (2007) T-helper 1 and 2 serum cytokine assay in chronic opioid addicts. Eur Cytokine Netw 18(4):210–214

Bar-Yosef S, Melamed R, Page GG, Shakhar G, Shakhar K, Ben-Eliyahu S (2001) Attenuation of the tumor-promoting effect of surgery by spinal blockade in rats. Anesthesiology 94(6):1066–1073

Börner C, Kraus J, Bedini A, Schraven B, Höllt V (2008) T-cell receptor/CD28-mediated activation of human T lymphocytes induces expression of functional mu-opioid receptors. Mol Pharmacol 74(2):496–504

Börner C, Warnick B, Smida M, Hartig R, Lindquist JA, Schraven B, Höllt V, Kraus J (2009) Mechanisms of opioid-mediated inhibition of human T cell receptor signaling. J Immunol 183(2):882–889

Breslow JM, Monroy MA, Daly JM, Meissler JJ, Gaughan J, Adler MW, Eisenstein TK (2011) Morphine, but not trauma, sensitizes to systemic Acinetobacter baumannii infection. J Neuroimmune Pharmacol 6(4):551–565

Cai SW, Yang SZ, Gao J, Pan K, Chen JY, Wang YL, Wei LX, Dong JH (2011) Prognostic significance of mast cell count following curative resection for pancreatic ductal adenocarcinoma. Surgery 149(4):576–584

Campana G, Sarti D, Spampinato S, Raffaeli W (2010) Long-term intrathecal morphine and bupivacaine upregulate MOR gene expression in lymphocytes. Int Immunopharmacol 10(9):1149–1152

Choi Y, Chuang LF, Lam KM, Kung HF, Wang JM, Osburn BI, Chuang RY (1999) Inhibition of chemokine-induced chemotaxis of monkey leukocytes by mu-opioid receptor agonists. In Vivo 13(5):389–396

Clark JD, Shi X, Li X, Qiao Y, Liang D, Angst MS, Yeomans DC (2007) Morphine reduces local cytokine expression and neutrophil infiltration after incision. Mol Pain 3:28

Diaconu NC, Rummukainen J, Naukkarinen A, Mättö M, Harvima RJ, Pelkonen J, Harvima IT (2011) Mast cell chymase is present in uterine cervical carcinoma and it detaches viable and growing cervical squamous carcinoma cells from substratum in vitro. Arch Dermatol Res 303(7):499–512

Ecimovic P, Murray D, Doran P, McDonald J, Lambert DG, Buggy DJ (2011) Direct effect of morphine on breast cancer cell function in vitro: role of the NET1 gene. Br J Anaesth 107(6):916–923

Fecho K, Manning EL, Maixner W, Schmitt CP (2007) Effects of carrageenan and morphine on acute inflammation and pain in Lewis and Fischer rats. Brain Behav Immun 21(1):68–78

Franchi S, Panerai AE, Sacerdote P (2007) Buprenorphine ameliorates the effect of surgery on hypothalamus-pituitary-adrenal axis, natural killer cell activity and metastatic colonization in rats in comparison with morphine or fentanyl treatment. Brain Behav Immun 21(6):767–774

Freier DO, Fuchs BA (1993) Morphine-induced alterations in thymocyte subpopulations of B6C3F1 mice. J Pharmacol Exp Ther 265(1):81–88

Fuggetta MP, Di Francesco P, Falchetti R, Cottarelli A, Rossi L, Tricarico M, Lanzilli G (2005) Effect of morphine on cell-mediated immune responses of human lymphocytes against allogeneic malignant cells. J Exp Clin Cancer Res 24(2):255–263

Gaspani L, Bianchi M, Limiroli E, Panerai AE, Sacerdote P (2002) The analgesic drug tramadol prevents the effect of surgery on natural killer cell activity and metastatic colonization in rats. J Neuroimmunol 129(1–2):18–24

Gordon EM, Myers C, Blumer J (2004) In vitro evaluation of the potential role of sulfite radical in morphine-associated histamine release. BMC Pharmacol 4:21

Greeneltch KM, Kelly-Welch AE, Shi Y, Keegan AD (2005) Chronic morphine treatment promotes specific Th2 cytokine production by murine T cells in vitro via a Fas/Fas ligand-dependent mechanism. J Immunol 175(8):4999–5005

Gregory AD, Houghton AM (2011) Tumor-associated neutrophils: new targets for cancer therapy. Cancer Res 71(7):2411–2416

Güttler K, Sabatowski R (2008) Differential therapeutic aspects of analgesia with oral sustained-release strong opioids: application intervals, metabolism and immunosuppression. Schmerz 22(5): 562, 564–568, 570.

Harari Y, Weisbrodt NW, Moody FG (2006) The effect of morphine on mast cell-mediated mucosal permeability. Surgery 139(1):54–60

Hatsukari I, Hitosugi N, Dinda A, Singhal PC (2006) Morphine modulates monocyte-macrophage conversion phase. Cell Immunol 239(1):41–48

Hatsukari I, Hitosugi N, Ohno R, Hashimoto K, Nakamura S, Satoh K, Nagasaka H, Matsumoto I, Sakagami H (2007) Induction of apoptosis by morphine in human tumor cell lines in vitro. Anticancer Res 27(2):857–864

Hu S, Chao CC, Hegg CC, Thayer S, Peterson PK (2000) Morphine inhibits human microglial cell production of, and migration towards, RANTES. J Psychopharmacol 14(3):238–243

Kalra M, Rao N, Rehman F, Tippu S, Arora A, Nanda K (2011) The role of mast cells on angiogenesis in oral squamous cell carcinoma. Med Oral Patol Oral Cir Bucal 17(2):e190-6. doi:10.4317/medoral.17395

Levy EM, Roberti MP, Mordoh J (2011) Natural killer cells in human cancer: from biological functions to clinical applications. J Biomed Biotechnol 2011:676198

Lewis C, Murdoch C (2005) Macrophage responses to hypoxia: implications for tumor progression and anti-cancer therapies. Am J Pathol 167:627–635

Li W, Tang HZ, Jiang YB, Xu MX (2003) Influence of different doses of fentanyl on T-lymphocyte subpopulations and natural killer cells of patients with esophageal tumor during preoperation and postoperation. Ai Zheng 22(6):634–636

Liang-Suo J, Gomez-Flores R, Weber RJ (2002) Immunosuppression induced by central action of morphine is not blocked by mifepristone (RU 486). Life Sci 71(22):2595–2602

Liao W, Lin JX, Leonard WJ (2011) IL-2 family cytokines: new insights into the complex roles of IL-2 as a broad regulator of T helper cell differentiation. Curr Opin Immunol 23(5):598–604

Liu Z, Gao F, Tian Y (2006) Effects of morphine, fentanyl and tramadol on human immune response. J Huazhong Univ Sci Technolog Med Sci 26(4):478–481
Madera-Salcedo IK, Cruz SL, Gonzalez-Espinosa C (2011) Morphine decreases early peritoneal innate immunity responses in Swiss-Webster and C57BL6/J mice through the inhibition of mast cell TNF-α release. J Neuroimmunol 232(1–2):101–107
Malik AA, Radhakrishnan N, Reddy K, Smith AD, Singhal PC (2002) Morphine-induced macrophage apoptosis modulates migration of macrophages: use of in vitro model of urinary tract infection. J Endourol 16(8):605–610
Maltby S, Freeman S, Gold MJ, Baker JH, Minchinton AI, Gold MR, Roskelley CD, McNagny KM (2011) Opposing roles for CD34 in B16 melanoma tumor growth alter early stage vasculature and late stage immune cell infiltration. PLoS One 6(4):e18160
Martin JL, Charboneau R, Barke RA, Roy S (2010) Chronic morphine treatment inhibits LPS-induced angiogenesis: implications in wound healing. Cell Immunol 265(2):139–145
Miller ST, Barney NP, Gamache DA, Spellman JM, Yanni JM (1997) Secretory response of mast cells contained in monodispersed human choroidal preparations. Int Arch Allergy Immunol 114(2):139–143
Miyagi T, Chuang LF, Lam KM, Kung H, Wang JM, Osburn BI, Chuang RY (2000) Opioids suppress chemokine-mediated migration of monkey neutrophils and monocytes – an instant response. Immunopharmacology 47(1):53–62
Mojadadi S, Jamali A, Khansarinejad B, Soleimanjahi H, Bamdad T (2009) Acute morphine administration reduces cell-mediated immunity and induces reactivation of latent herpes simplex virus type 1 in BALB/c mice. Cell Mol Immunol 6(2):111–116
Movahedi K, Guilliams M, Van den Bossche J, Van den Bergh R, Gysemans C, Beschin A, De Baetselier P, Van Ginderachter JA (2008) Identification of discrete tumor-induced myeloid-derived suppressor cell subpopulations with distinct T cell-suppressive activity. Blood 111:4233–4244
Murdoch C, Muthana M, Coffelt SB, Lewis CE (2008) The role of myeloid cells in the promotion of tumour angiogenesis. Nat Rev Cancer 8(8):618–631 (Review)
Ohara T, Itoh T, Takahashi M (2005) Immunosuppression by morphine-induced lymphocyte apoptosis: is it a real issue? Anesth Analg 101(4):1117–1122
Pan PY, Wang GX, Yin B, Ozao J, Ku T, Divino CM, Chen SH (2008) Reversion of immune tolerance in advanced malignancy: modulation of myeloid-derived suppressor cell development by blockade of stem-cell factor function. Blood 111:219–228
Pansrikaew P, Cheewakriangkrai C, Taweevisit M, Khunamornpong S, Siriaunkgul S (2010) Correlation of mast cell density, tumor angiogenesis, and clinical outcomes in patients with endometrioid endometrial cancer. Asian Pac J Cancer Prev 11(3):623–626
Pergolizzi JV Jr, Mercadante S, Echaburu AV, Van den Eynden B, Fragoso RM, Mordarski S, Lybaert W, Beniak J, Orońska A, Slama O (2009) The role of transdermal buprenorphine in the treatment of cancer pain: an expert panel consensus. Curr Med Res Opin 25(6):1517–1528
Rahim RT, Meissler JJ Jr, Adler MW, Eisenstein TK (2005) Splenic macrophages and B cells mediate immunosuppression following abrupt withdrawal from morphine. J Leukoc Biol 78(6):1185–1191
Ribatti D, Guidolin D, Marzullo A, Nico B, Annese T, Benagiano V, Crivellato E (2010) Mast cells and angiogenesis in gastric carcinoma. Int J Exp Pathol 91(4):350–356
Risdahl JM, Huether MJ, Gustafson KV, Molitor TW (1995) Morphine alteration of histamine release in vivo. Adv Exp Med Biol 373:161–168
Roy S, Wang J, Charboneau R, Loh HH, Barke RA (2005) Morphine induces CD4+ T cell IL-4 expression through an adenylyl cyclase mechanism independent of the protein kinase A pathway. J Immunol 175(10):6361–6367
Roy S, Ninkovic J, Banerjee S, Charboneau RG, Das S, Dutta R, Kirchner VA, Koodie L, Ma J, Meng J, Barke RA (2011) Opioid drug abuse and modulation of immune function: consequences in the susceptibility to opportunistic infections. J Neuroimmune Pharmacol 6(4):442–465
Sedqi M, Roy S, Ramakrishnan S, Elde R, Loh H (1995) Complementary DNA cloning of a mu-opioid receptor from rat peritoneal macrophages. Biochem Biophys Res Commun 209:563–574
Sheen CH, Schleimer RP, Kulka M (2007) Codeine induces human mast cell chemokine and cytokine production: involvement of G-protein activation. Allergy 62(5):532–538

Shirzad H, Shahrani M, Rafieian-Kopaei M (2009) Comparison of morphine and tramadol effects on phagocytic activity of mice peritoneal phagocytes in vivo. Int Immunopharmacol 9(7–8):968–970
Stankiewicz E, Wypasek E, Plytycz B (2004) Mast cells are responsible for the lack of anti-inflammatory effects of morphine in CBA mice. Mediat Inflamm 13(5–6):365–368
Stefano GB, Cadet P, Fimiani C, Magazine HI (2001) Morphine stimulates iNOS expression via a rebound from inhibition in human macrophages: nitric oxide involvement. Int J Immunopathol Pharmacol 14(3):129–138
Tadmor T, Attias D, Polliack A (2011) Myeloid-derived suppressor cells – their role in haemato-oncological malignancies and other cancers and possible implications for therapy. Br J Haematol 153(5):557–567
Talmadge JE (2011) Immune cell infiltration of primary and metastatic lesions: mechanisms and clinical impact. Semin Cancer Biol 21(2):131–138
Tegeder I, Grösch S, Schmidtko A, Häussler A, Schmidt H, Niederberger E, Scholich K, Geisslinger G (2003) G protein-independent G1 cell cycle block and apoptosis with morphine in adenocarcinoma cells: involvement of p53 phosphorylation. Cancer Res 63(8):1846–1852
Vasievich EA, Huang L (2011) The suppressive tumor microenvironment: a challenge in cancer immunotherapy. Mol Pharm 8(3):635–641
Wang HW, Joyce JA (2010) Alternative activation of tumor-associated macrophages by IL-4: priming for protumoral functions. Cell Cycle 9(24):4824–4835
Wang J, Barke RA, Charboneau R, Roy S (2005) Morphine impairs host innate immune response and increases susceptibility to Streptococcus pneumoniae lung infection. J Immunol 174(1):426–434
Wang J, Barke RA, Roy S (2007) Transcriptional and epigenetic regulation of interleukin-2 gene in activated T cells by morphine. J Biol Chem 282(10):7164–7171
Wang J, Charboneau R, Balasubramanian S, Barke RA, Loh HH, Roy S (2002) The immunosuppressive effects of chronic morphine treatment are partially dependent on corticosterone and mediated by the mu-opioid receptor. J Leukoc Biol 71(5):782–790
Wang ZY, Wang CQ, Yang JJ, Sun J, Huang YH, Tang QF, Qian YN (2006) Which has the least immunity depression during postoperative analgesia–morphine, tramadol, or tramadol with lornoxicam? Clin Chim Acta 369(1):40–45
Weed MR, Carruth LM, Adams RJ, Ator NA, Hienz RD (2006) Morphine withdrawal dramatically reduces lymphocytes in morphine-dependent macaques. J Neuroimmune Pharmacol 1(3):250–259
Welters ID, Menzebach A, Goumon Y, Cadet P, Menges T, Hughes TK, Hempelmann G, Stefano GB (2000a) Morphine inhibits NF-kappaB nuclear binding in human neutrophils and monocytes by a nitric oxide-dependent mechanism. Anesthesiology 92(6):1677–1684
Welters ID, Menzebach A, Goumon Y, Langefeld TW, Teschemacher H, Hempelmann G, Stefano GB (2000b) Morphine suppresses complement receptor expression, phagocytosis, and respiratory burst in neutrophils by a nitric oxide and mu(3) opiate receptor-dependent mechanism. J Neuroimmunol 111(1–2):139–145
Wypasek E, Natorska J, Stankiewicz E, Kolaczkowska E (2011) Morphine-modulated mast cell migration and proliferation during early stages of zymosan-induced peritonitis in CBA mice. Folia Biol (Krakow) 59(3–4):99–106
Xia Q, Wu XJ, Zhou Q, Jing-Zeng HJH, Pan ZZ, Zhang XS (2011) No relationship between the distribution of mast cells and the survival of stage IIIB colon cancer patients. J Transl Med 9(9):88
Xiang M, Gu Y, Zhao F, Lu H, Chen S, Yin L (2010) Mast cell tryptase promotes breast cancer migration and invasion. Oncol Rep 23(3):615–619
Ye XZ, Yu SC, Bian XW (2010) Contribution of myeloid-derived suppressor cells to tumor-induced immune suppression, angiogenesis, invasion and metastasis. J Genet Genomics 37(7):423–430
Yin D, Mufson RA, Wang R, Shi Y (1999) Fas-mediated cell death promoted by opioids. Nature 397(6716):218
Yin D, Woodruff M, Zhang Y, Whaley S, Miao J, Ferslew K, Zhao J, Stuart C (2006) Morphine promotes Jurkat cell apoptosis through pro-apoptotic FADD/P53 and anti-apoptotic PI3K/Akt/NF-kappaB pathways. J Neuroimmunol 174(1–2):101–107
Yossuck P, Nightengale BJ, Fortney JE, Gibson LF (2008) Effect of morphine sulfate on neonatal neutrophil chemotaxis. Clin J Pain 24(1):76–82

# Chapter 4
# Opioid Regulation of Vascular Integrity

**Frances E. Lennon and Patrick A. Singleton**

**Abstract** Endothelial barrier integrity is crucial to the maintenance of vascular homeostasis. Dysfunction of the vascular endothelial barrier is associated with a wide range of pathologies including atherosclerosis, stroke, inflammatory disorders, acute lung injury, multiple sclerosis, cancer and diabetes mellitus. Although opioids are widely used during the treatment of many classes of disease and injury, the interaction of opioids with the endothelial barrier is not well understood. This chapter reviews what is currently known about opioid regulation of barrier integrity and in particular its effect on endothelial permeability, angiogenesis and inflammation. The role of mu opioid receptor activation, receptor tyrosine kinase transactivation and downstream signaling pathways are discussed. Further the role of mu opioid receptor antagonists as potential therapeutic agents in endothelial barrier dysfunction is examined.

**Keywords** Angiogenesis • Endothelial barrier • Inflammation • Signaling • Opioids • Opioid receptor antagonists • Vascular integrity

F.E. Lennon
Department of Medicine, Section of Pulmonary and Critical Care,
Pritzker School of Medicine, The University of Chicago,
5841 South Maryland Avenue, MC 6076, I-503C, Chicago, IL 60637, USA
e-mail: franlen@gmail.com

P.A. Singleton (✉)
Department of Medicine, Section of Pulmonary and Critical Care,
Pritzker School of Medicine, The University of Chicago,
5841 South Maryland Avenue, MC 6076, I-503C, Chicago, IL 60637, USA

Department of Anesthesia and Critical Care, Pritzker School of Medicine,
The University of Chicago, 5841 South Maryland Avenue,
MC 6076, I-503C, Chicago, IL 60637, USA
e-mail: psinglet@medicine.bsd.uchicago.edu

M.-O. Parat (ed.), *Morphine and Metastasis*, DOI 10.1007/978-94-007-5678-6_4, 

## Abbreviations

| | |
|---|---|
| DAMGO | [D-Ala2, N-MePhe4, Gly-ol]-enkephalin |
| cAMP | adenosine 3′ 5′-cyclic monophosphate |
| AC | adenylate cyclase |
| BBB | blood–brain-barrier |
| CAM | chick chorioallantonic model |
| ECAM | endothelial cell adhesion molecule |
| EGFR | epidermal growth factor receptor |
| GPCRs | G-protein coupled receptors |
| GEFs | guanine nucleotide exchange factors |
| GTPases | guanosine triphosphatases |
| HA | hyaluronan |
| HIF | hypoxia-inducible factor |
| IGFR | insulin-like growth factor receptor |
| ICAM-1 | intercellular adhesion molecule 1 |
| IL-1 | interleukin-1 |
| JAM-2 | junctional adhesion molecule 2 |
| JAMs | junctional adhesion molecules |
| LPS | lipopolysaccharide |
| MNTX | methylnaltrexone |
| MAPK | mitogen-activated protein kinase |
| MLC | myosin light chain |
| MLCK | myosin-light chain kinase |
| PDGF | platelet-derived growth factor |
| PKA | protein kinase A |
| Akt | protein kinase B |
| RhoA | Ras homolog gene family, member A |
| RTKs | receptor tyrosine kinases |
| S1P | sphingosine-1-phosphate |
| SH3 | SRC Homology 3 |
| SIRS | systemic inflammatory response syndrome |
| VCAM | Vascular cell adhesion molecule |
| VEGF | vascular endothelial growth factor |
| VEGFR | Vascular endothelial growth factor receptor |
| VE-cadherin | Vascular-endothelial cadherin |
| ZO | zona occludens |

## 4.1 Introduction

Vascular integrity is a fundamental process which balances a variety of factors to maintain blood vessel continuity. This balance is maintained via cell–cell and cell–matrix contacts and through hormonal and chemokine signaling pathways. A number of different cell types including endothelial, smooth muscle cells and pericytes all contribute to maintaining vascular integrity. Disruption of vascular integrity is associated with a number of serious pathologies including atherosclerosis, stroke, inflammatory disorders, acute lung injury, multiple sclerosis, cancer and diabetes (Miano and Berk 2006; Yuan and Rigor 2010).

## 4.2 Vascular Endothelium

The vascular endothelium, which lines the inner surface of blood vessels, acts as a selectively permeable barrier to regulate the movement of liquid and solutes between blood and the surrounding tissue, particularly in the microvasculature (Curry and Adamson 2010; Dejana et al. 2009b; Vandenbroucke et al. 2008; Yuan and Rigor 2010). The semi-permeable nature of the endothelium allows plasma fluid, nutrients and even cells to move out of the blood and into the tissues while metabolic products may be taken up by the circulation (Yuan and Rigor 2010). This exchange, between the blood and the tissues is vital for organ function and tissue viability by maintaining fluid and metabolic homeostasis. Vascular permeability is mediated via two pathways known as the paracellular (via gaps between the endothelial cells) and transcellular (via vesicle transport through the cell body) pathways (Dejana et al. 2009b). Vascular barrier function is dependent on the integrity of the endothelial cell layer. Disruption or dysregulation of the endothelial layer can lead to altered permeability resulting in leakage of fluid, solutes and proteins from the blood into the underlying tissue resulting in edema. This in turn can lead to an increase in interstitial pressure and disrupt tissue perfusion and organ function. Vascular leak and edema can also stimulate increased leukocyte transendothelial migration and infiltration into the tissue. Altered permeability may even lead to the rupture of the vessel and clot formation (Dejana et al. 2009b). Dysregulation of endothelial barrier function can occur in a wide range of human pathophysiologies including inflammation, sepsis, acute lung injury/acute respiratory distress syndrome, trauma, ischemia/reperfusion injury, metastatic tumor development and diabetes mellitus.

### *4.2.1 Adherens Junctions*

Vascular barrier function is dependent on endothelial cell–cell contacts. Endothelial cells have three different types of cell–cell junctional complexes, including adherens junctions, tight junctions and gap junctions (Dejana et al. 2009b). Adherens junctions are the predominant junction type in the endothelium. Their main function is to initiate and maintain cell–cell contact. Vascular-endothelial (VE)-cadherin is believed to be the most important protein in the adherens junction, both functionally and from a regulatory standpoint. VE-cadherin is a transmembrane protein, consisting of 5-cadherin-like repeats that can associate homotypically with VE-cadherin in the adjoining cell in a $Ca^{2+}$ dependent manner (Vandenbroucke et al. 2008). VE-cadherin

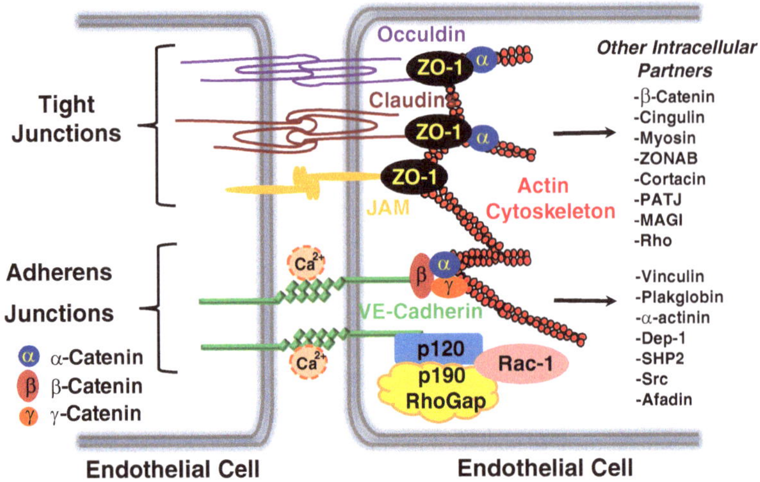


**Fig. 4.1** Illustration of endothelial cell–cell contacts. Tight junctions and adherens junctions are involved in the regulation of cell–cell contacts. In tight junctions, adhesion is mediated by homotypic binding of claudins, occludins and junctional adhesion molecules (JAMs). Intracellularly, these proteins connect to the actin cytoskeleton via ZO-1, α-catenin and a host of other associated signaling proteins. VE-Cadherin is the key component of adherens junctions. It associates with the actin cytoskeleton via α, β, γ-catenins and to RhoGAP via p120-catenin. Other actin-binding proteins and signaling proteins associated with adherens junctions are listed above. A more complete review of the structure and regulation of adherens and tight junctions can be found in the following (Dejana et al. 2009a; Martin and Jiang 2009; Vandenbroucke et al. 2008; Yuan and Rigor 2010)

in turn binds to a number of intracellular proteins including p120-catenin and β-catenin. These interactions are required to maintain junctional stability. p120-catenin acts as a scaffold protein to link VE-cadherin with a number of downstream signaling pathways including kinases, phosphatases and Rho guanosine triphosphatases (GTPases). β-catenin links VE-cadherin with the actin cytoskeleton via α-catenin. The dynamic interaction between VE-cadherins, the actin cytoskeleton and downstream signaling pathways is crucial to the regulation of vascular integrity and permeability (Fig. 4.1).

### *4.2.2 Tight Junctions*

Tight junctions, although considerably less prevalent in the endothelium that adherens junctions, are essential in maintaining vascular barrier function. They are involved in regulating paracellular permeability although their exact role is less well understood than adherens junctions. Tight junctions act to demarcate the basalolateral and apical regions of the cell as they prevent diffusion of plasma membrane lipids and proteins thereby establishing and maintaining cell polarity (Dejana et al. 2009b; Martin and Jiang 2009; Vandenbroucke et al. 2008; Yuan and Rigor 2010). Tight junctions are formed by homotypic adhesion of occludin, claudins and junctional adhesion molecules (JAMs). These transmembrane proteins are in turn bound by zona occludens (ZO)-1,-2 and α-catenin which connect them to the cytoskeleton (Fig. 4.1). ZO-1 and ZO-2 can also act a signaling or scaffold molecule as they contain a PDZ domain, a guanylate kinase domain and a SRC homology 3 (SH3) domain (Yuan and Rigor 2010).

### *4.2.3 Other Junctional and Adhesion Complexes*

Gap junctions are found mostly in larger vessels and are involved in cell–cell communication between adjoining endothelial cells and endothelial and smooth muscle cells. They are not believed to play a direct role in regulating vascular function (Dejana et al. 2009b; Yuan and Rigor 2010).

Focal adhesions, which are contacts between the underlying basement matrix and the endothelial cell, also contribute to barrier integrity. These contacts are vital to endothelial cell function and viability and disruption of these integrin mediated contacts has been shown to increase endothelial permeability (Yuan and Rigor 2010). Vascular permeability is regulated via endothelial activation or stimulation. Agents that induce cortical actin formation required for endothelial barrier enhancement include sphingosine-1-phosphate (S1P) (Singleton et al. 2005), high molecular weight hyaluronic acid (HA) (Singleton et al. 2006a), angiopoetin-1 (Lee and Liles 2011), Adenosine 3′ 5′-cyclic monophosphate (cAMP) (Moore et al. 1998) and iloprost (Birukova et al. 2010). A number of barrier disruptive (permeability increasing) agents that lead to actin stress fiber formation includes thrombin, vascular endothelial growth factor (VEGF), lipopolysaccharide (LPS), low molecular weight hyaluronic acid (HA) and histamine (Surapisitchat and Beavo 2011).

Vascular integrity may be disrupted during angiogenic remodeling, wound healing, inflammation and by immune or tumor cell extravasation. During the initial phases of angiogenesis, endothelial cells must detach themselves from the surrounding cells and the underlying matrix in order to migrate and proliferate into the surrounding tissue and form new blood vessels. During this stage there is an increase in vascular permeability. Inflammatory mediators released during immune cell recruitment, adhesion and extravasation can also stimulate an increase in vascular permeability. In most pathophysiological states the paracellular pathway (between the cells) is responsible for the increased leakage of fluid and proteins from the blood (Yuan and Rigor 2010).

## 4.3 Opioids and Vascular Integrity

Opiate receptors (μ, δ, and κ) are members of the G-protein coupled class of seven-pass transmembrane receptors. The mu opioid receptor couples to the $G_{i/o}$ inhibitory subunit, which upon ligand binding dissociates into its $G_\alpha$ and $G_{\beta\gamma}$ subunits which in turn act on various intracellular signaling pathways (Al-Hasani and Bruchas 2011;

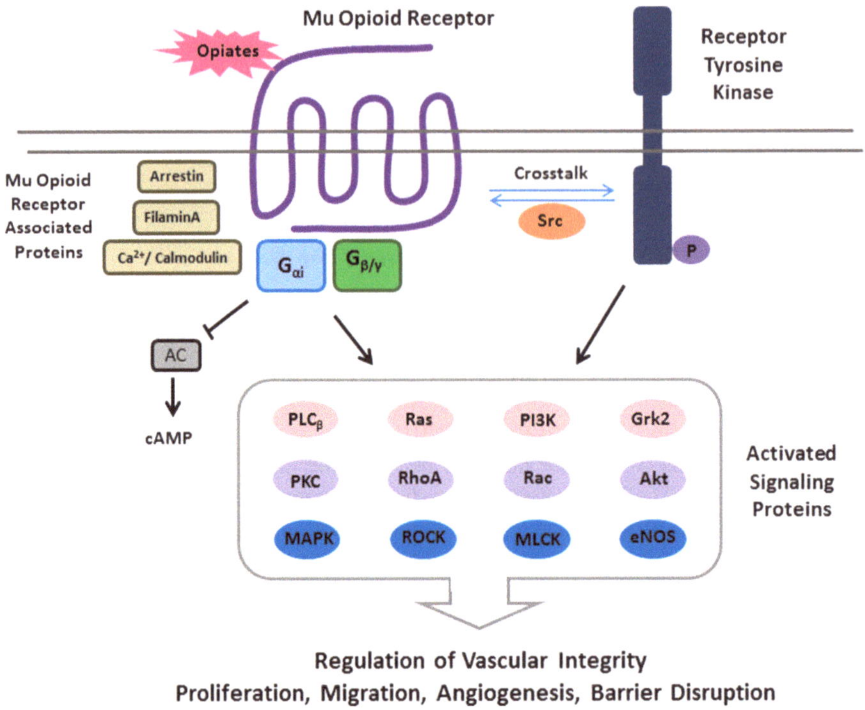


**Fig. 4.2** Mu opioid receptor signaling in endothelial cells. The mu opioid receptor couples to $G_{\alpha i}$/$G_{\beta\gamma}$ G-protein subunits which dissociate following acute opioid activation. $G_{\alpha i}$ inhibits adenylate cyclase activity, while $G_{\beta\gamma}$ is involved in the activation of other downstream signaling pathways including Src which may be involved in transactivation of receptor tyrosine kinases. Other mu opioid receptor-associated proteins, including filamin A, arrestin and calmodulin, modulate receptor activation/deactivation, recycling and degradation. Activation of downstream signaling pathways including RhoA, PI3K, and MAPKs regulate endothelial barrier integrity via changes in endothelial cell permeability which can lead to altered proliferation, migration and angiogenesis. A more complete review of mu opioid receptor signaling pathways and associated proteins can be found in the following (Al-Hasani and Bruchas 2011; Milligan 2005; Tegeder and Geisslinger 2004; Waters et al. 2004)

Tegeder and Geisslinger 2004). A number of other proteins can also associate with the mu-opioid receptor to further modulate its activity including calmodulin, filamin A and β-arrestin (Milligan 2005). G-protein coupled receptors (GPCRs), including the mu opioid receptor can also stimulate transactivation of receptor tyrosine kinases (RTKs), including epidermal growth factor receptor (EGFR), Insulin-like growth factor receptor (IGFR) and Vascular endothelial growth factor receptor (VEGFR) and mulitple levels of signal integration are believed to exist between the two receptor systems (Fujioka et al. 2011; Singleton et al. 2006b; Waters et al. 2004). A generalized overview of mu opioid receptor signaling and RTK transactivation in endothelial cells is illustrated in Fig. 4.2.

### 4.3.1 Endothelial Barrier Permeability

cAMP is a key regulator of endothelial barrier permeability. It has been shown to prevent or reverse permeability-induced pulmonary edema in numerous animal models (Moore et al. 1998). The barrier-enhancing effects of cAMP are mediated largely by the actions of protein kinase A (PKA). PKA enhances barrier function by inhibiting activation of RhoA and directly and indirectly inhibiting myosin light chain (MLC) phosphorylation. This inhibits cell contraction and helps to stabilize cell–cell contacts. Opioid receptor coupling and signaling via $G_{\alpha i}$ inhibitory subunits, lead to inhibition of adenylate cyclase (AC) and decreased cAMP production (Al-Hasani and Bruchas 2011; Sharma et al. 1975). Opioid-induced inhibition of cAMP production may therefore result in decreased barrier function. Morphine and DAMGO ([D-Ala2, N-MePhe4, Gly-ol]-enkephalin, a synthetic opioid peptide) have been shown to decrease pulmonary microvascular endothelial cell barrier function *in vitro* (Singleton et al. 2006b). This increase in permeability can be blocked by pretreatment of the cells with the mu opioid receptor antagonist methylnaltrexone (MNTX). Treatment with DAMGO and morphine stimulated increased $S1P_3$ receptor threonine phosphorylation. $S1P_3$ receptor activation is associated with endothelial barrier disruptive effects and activates Ras homolog gene family, member A (RhoA)-mediated signaling (Singleton et al. 2006a; Waeber et al. 2004). Further investigation revealed that DAMGO and morphine both stimulate RhoA signaling via recruitment of the Rho guanine nucleotide exchange factor (GEF) p115 to the $S1P_3$ receptor. Treatment with mu opioid receptor agonists induces transactivation of the $S1P_3$ receptor. Pretreatment with MNTX inhibits this transactivation reaction and preserves endothelial barrier function (Singleton et al. 2007). A number of clinical case reports have indicated that exposure to opiates can lead to the development of peripheral and in some cases pulmonary edema (Gardner-Nix 2002; Ruan et al. 2008) which are resolved following cessation of the opioid treatment.

Contrary to the previous discussed studies, morphine has been reported to attenuate microvascular hyperpermeability following hemorrhagic shock in rats. In a study by Puana et al., administration of morphine sulfate following hemorrhagic shock decreases vascular leak in a PKA dependent manner via inhibition of Raf-1 and mitogen-activated protein kinase (MAPK) activity (Puana et al. 2008).

Chronic exposure to opioids is associated with an increase in cAMP levels (Al-Hasani and Bruchas 2011). This increase in cAMP production may be due to a switch from $G_{\alpha i}$ inhibitory signaling to the AC stimulatory $G_{\beta\gamma}$ signaling and may be involved in the development of opioid tolerance (Gintzler and Chakrabarti 2006). The effect of acute or chronic opioid exposure on AC activity may also be isoform specific (Schallmach et al. 2006). AC isoforms I, V, VI and VII are inhibited by acute opioid exposure while AC isoforms II, IV and VII are stimulated following opioid exposure (Schallmach et al. 2006). This ability to switch from cAMP inhibiting (barrier disruptive) to cAMP producing (a barrier enhancing) a signaling pathways can help to explain the apparently contradictory reports of morphine as a endothelial barrier disruptive or inhibitory agent.

### *4.3.2 The Blood–Brain Barrier*

A specialized example of endothelial vascular integrity is demonstrated in the blood–brain-barrier (BBB). The BBB is formed by interaction between endothelial cells and glial cells. Brain endothelial cells have distinct structural and functional properties compared to other microvascular endothelial cells. While they do possess adherens junctions similar to other endothelial cells, they have very high resistance tight junctions, are not fenestrated and exhibit low pinocytotic activity. Transport of necessary nutrients into the brain and export of toxic metabolites is regulated by membrane transport proteins and receptors including glucose transporters, insulin and transferrin receptors and ATP-binding cassette transporters (Abbott et al. 2010; Hawkins and Davis 2005; Paolinelli et al. 2011). The BBB is therefore a very closely regulated and restrictive barrier between the circulating blood and the central nervous system. Disruption of the BBB is recognized as a critical factor in a growing number of human pathologies including hypoxia/ischemia stroke, multiple sclerosis, Parkinson's disease, Alzheimer's disease and HIV/AIDS (Abbott et al. 2010; Hawkins and Davis 2005; Mahajan et al. 2008). A number of recent studies suggest that increasing opiate use for pain management (or opiate abuse) may be a contributing factor for increased neuroinflammation and may exacerbate some neuropathologies (Wen et al. 2011). ZO-1, a key regulator of tight junction function, is down regulated in brain-derived endothelial microvascular cells in response to morphine (μM concentration, 3–24 h) treatment (Wen et al. 2011). Morphine also stimulated platelet-derived growth factor (PDGF)-B expression and phosphorylation of p44/p42 MAPK, p38 and protein kinase B (Akt), in these cells. Endothelial barrier function is compromised following morphine treatment leading to an increase in endothelial permeability (Chang et al. 2001; Wen et al. 2011). Barrier function could be preserved however by pre-treating the cells with naltrexone, an opioid receptor antagonist, or a PDGF-B neutralizing antibody (Wen et al. 2011). Morphine treatment has also been reported to increase the expression of the adhesion molecules Intercellular Adhesion Molecule 1 (ICAM-1), Vascular cell adhesion molecule (VCAM) and endothelial cell adhesion molecule (ECAM) in brain microvascular endothelial cells (Chang et al. 2001).

Studies have shown that HIV-1 patients who abuse opiates are at greater risk of developing neurological complications (Donahoe and Vlahov 1998). This has led to a number of studies investigating the possible interaction between opiates, HIV-1 and the BBB. Treatment of brain-derived endothelial cells with a combination of morphine (μM) and HIV-1 tat significantly altered expression of a number of tight junction-associated genes including ZO-1, occludin and junctional adhesion molecule 2 (JAM-2). Myosin-light chain kinase (MLCK), another protein involved in regulating endothelial permeability, showed synergistic increases in expression following incubation with a combination of morphine and tat when compared to cells treated with either tat or morphine alone (Mahajan et al. 2008). An *in vitro* BBB model using a co-culture of brain-derived endothelial cells and astrocytes also demonstrates synergistic increases in permeability when treated with a combination of morphine and tat (Mahajan et al. 2008). Chronic exposure to morphine *in vivo* is associated with changes in BBB gene expression in rats although no increase in BBB permeability was detected (Yousif et al. 2008). An increase in BBB permeability has been observed in a rodent model of morphine withdrawal. In this model Sprague–Dawley rats were given daily injections of morphine (10 mg/kg i.p.) for 12 consecutive days, morphine administration was then stopped and withdrawal symptoms were noted daily for 72 h. Increased BBB permeability (as measured by Evans Blue tracer or radio-labelled iodine leakage) is significantly increased at 24 and 48 h following morphine withdrawal.

### *4.3.3 Endothelial Cell Proliferation*

Although mainly expressed on neurons, other cells types including endothelial, epithelial, smooth muscle and immune cells can also express the mu opioid receptor. Morphine has been shown to stimulate endothelial cell proliferation at low concentrations (nM to μM range) but may conversely stimulate apoptosis and decrease cell viability at higher concentrations (μM to mM range) using *in vitro* assays (Leo et al. 2009; Liu et al. 2004). Low concentrations of morphine (100 nM) stimulate endothelial cell migration and transactivate the VEGR2 *in vitro* (Singleton et al. 2006b). This increase in proliferation may be mediated in part via activation of MAPKs p44/p42 as it may be blocked by the MAPK pathway inhibitor PD98059 (Leo et al. 2009). In the HEK293 cell line mu opioid receptor stimulated activation of MAPKs was shown to be mediated via a direct interaction with calmodulin resulting in the transactivation of the EGF receptor, ultimately resulting in MAPK activation (Belcheva et al. 2001). Increased Src phosphorylation is also observed in endothelial cells following incubation with morphine or DAMGO (Singleton et al. 2006b). Silencing of Src blocks the effects of opioid activation on VEGFR phosphorylation and inhibits opioid-induced endothelial cell proliferation and migration. It has also been reported that Src phosphorylation can act as a switch which alters mu opioid receptor signaling from an inhibitory to a stimulatory signal (Zhang et al. 2009). Some differences in the response of endothelial cells to morphine stimulation have been reported relating to the source of the endothelial cells i.e. macrovascular versus microvascular cells. Endogeneous opioids endomorphin-1,-2 and deltorphin-I can stimulate endothelial cell proliferation *in vitro* (Dai et al. 2010).

### *4.3.4 Angiogenesis*

Morphine and endogenous opioids have been shown to modulate angiogenesis both *in vitro* and *in vivo*. A number of groups demonstrated that morphine can stimulate angiogenesis. *In vitro*, morphine (1 μM) stimulates increased endothelial tube formation on matrigel, although cytotoxicity was observed at higher concentrations (>100 μM).

*In vivo* morphine (10 μM in matrigel plug) stimulates angiogenesis in a matrigel plug assay, while supraphysiological concentrations of morphine (10 mM) do not promote angiogenesis (Gupta et al. 2002). "Clinically relevant" doses of morphine (0.714 mg/kg/day) also stimulated breast tumor xenograft angiogenesis in this study. Interestingly, although co-administration of the mu-opioid receptor antagonist naloxone (10 μM naloxone in matrigel plug) did not inhibit morphine-induced angiogenesis in the matrigel plug assay, it did inhibit angiogenesis in the breast tumor xenograft. Naloxone-treated animals also had significantly smaller tumor volumes.

Clinically relevant doses of morphine (0.714 mg/kg/day per mouse, equivalent to 50 mg/day for a 70 kg human) stimulated tumor angiogenesis in a mouse breast cancer model. In this study, microvessel density was significantly increased ($p < 0.001$) in the tumors of mice who had received morphine (Ustun et al. 2011). The endogenous opioid peptides endomorphin-1,-2 and deltorphin I all stimulated increased blood vessel growth in a chick chorioallantonic model (CAM) of angiogenesis. In this model, the opioid peptides stimulate increased outgrowth of the smaller branch vessels, not just continued growth of the established blood vessels. This increase in angiogenesis is antagonized by co-administration of naloxone (Dai et al. 2008).

Disruption of the endothelial barrier during angiogenesis or even tumor surgery triggers dissemination of tumor cells into the vasculature facilitating metastatic spread of the disease (Le Guelte et al. 2011). It has been suggested that opioids, which contribute to this barrier disruption and are immune suppressive, can facilitate tumor cell entry into, or exit from, the vasculature (Singleton and Moss 2010). The role of morphine and other opioid analgesics in the spread of metastatic disease is a current topic of active research (Afsharimani et al. 2011; Snyder and Greenberg 2010).

However morphine has also been reported to inhibit angiogenesis in certain models. One study using Lewis lung carcinoma cells in a mouse matrigel plug model of tumor growth indicates that morphine suppresses tumor growth by inhibiting angiogenesis (Koodie et al. 2010). In this study, mice were implanted with morphine pellets (75 mg morphine) on day one along with the matrigel plug. On the final day (day 7) of the experiment the morphine concentration in plasma was measured as 300 ng/ml. The authors report that morphine suppresses hypoxia-induced p38 MAPK activation, which in turn decreases hypoxia-inducible factor (HIF)-1α expression. HIF-1α is a transcription factor that can regulate the expression of many genes involved in angiogenesis including VEGF. By inhibiting HIF-1α expression morphine could effectively suppress the tumor pro-angiogeneic response to hypoxia (Koodie et al. 2010).

Prolonged morphine exposure inhibits angiogenesis and wound healing in a mouse model (Lam et al. 2008). High doses of morphine (20 mg/kg/day) for 14 consecutive days, delivered via intraperitoneal injection, was shown to inhibit angiogenesis in a mouse matrigel plug assay. Delayed excisional wound healing was also observed in response to prolonged morphine exposure. Increased superoxide production was shown to occur in the tissue surrounding the wound of the morphine treated animals. In addition, morphine treatment decreases the numbers of circulating endothelial progenitor (CD34+/CD133+ mononuclear) cells (Lam et al. 2008).

### 4.3.5 *Inflammation and Sepsis*

Opioids are known to have inhibitory effects on the immune system. Acute and chronic opioid administration can affect both cellular and humoral immunity (Sacerdote 2006). Morphine suppresses lymphocyte trafficking and proliferation, inhibits antibody production and natural killer cell activity. Chronic opioid users have an increased susceptibility to bacterial infection (Ocasio et al. 2004). Disruption of vascular barrier function may also contribute to the compromised immune response. Sepsis is a severe bacterial infection which produces a systemic immune response in the patient. It occurs in more than 750,000 patients annually in the United States and is responsible for more that 210,000 deaths (Skrupky et al. 2011). Septic shock is the most severe form of sepsis and is the most common cause of death in the intensive care unit (Ocasio et al. 2004). Disruption of vascular barrier integrity and endothelial dysfunction play a key role in the pathogenesis of sepsis (Huet et al. 2011). Septic shock causes a dramatic decrease in blood pressure and the onset of disseminated intravascular coagulation (Ocasio et al. 2004). This drop in blood pressure and increased coagulation can lead to severe tissue damage and organ failure and is caused in part by increased vascular permeability. Morphine (10 μM) potentiates the barrier-disruptive effects of LPS on endothelial cells *in vitro* leading to increased endothelial permeability (Liu et al. 2004). Interleukin-1 (IL-1) is a pro-inflammatory cytokine secreted by cells in response to LPS/endotoxin. IL-1 up-regulates expression of the mu opioid receptor on endothelial cells and may further potentiate the effects of morphine on endothelial cells (Chang et al. 2001). Chronic morphine treatment, delivered via 75 mg morphine sulphate pellet implant, accelerates the progression of LPS-induced sepsis to septic shock in a rat model (Ocasio et al. 2004).

Endogenous morphine production is increased in response to inflammation and systemic infection, which may form part of the stress response and be an attempt by the body to maintain vascular homeostasis (Glattard et al. 2010). In a study of critically ill patients with varying degrees of systemic inflammatory response syndrome (SIRS), sepsis or septic shock, patients who develop sepsis or septic shock have significantly higher levels of serum morphine compared to SIRS patients. Morphine could not be detected in the serum of healthy controls (Glattard et al. 2010). However the low concentrations of morphine detected in the serum of sepsis patients (median concentration 2.00 ng/ml) are sufficient to inhibit the secretion of the pro-inflammatory IL-8 by neutrophils *in vitro* (Glattard et al. 2010).

## 4.4 Conclusion

Regulation of vascular integrity is a key factor in maintaining vascular homeostasis. Disruption or dysfunction of the endothelial barrier is implicated in a wide range of pathologies from acute lung injury to tumor metastasis (Fig. 4.3). The role of opiates

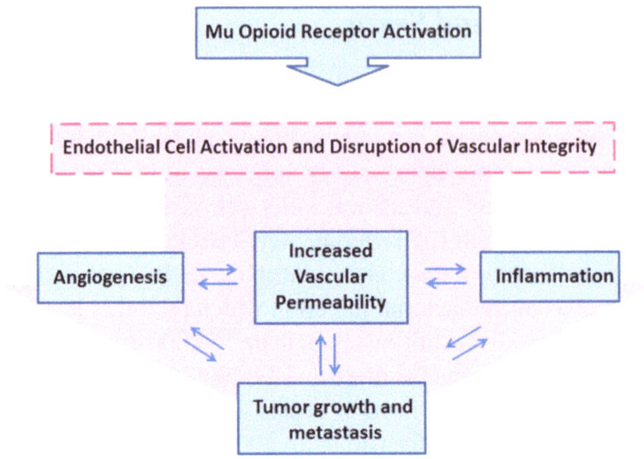


**Fig. 4.3** Opioids and vascular integrity. Schematic overview of the role of opioids in regulating vascular integrity. Opioid binding to the mu opioid receptor leads to endothelial cell activation and disruption of vascular integrity which can lead to altered vascular permeability, endothelial proliferation and angiogenesis. These changes can, in turn, modulate inflammatory responses, tumor growth and cancer metastatic

and mu opioid receptor signaling in endothelial barrier function is complex and is dependent not only on concentration but also on the length of exposure. Low doses of morphine (<μM) appear to stimulate increased endothelial barrier permeability and promote angiogenesis *in vivo*. Higher doses of morphine (>μM) have been reported to inhibit angiogenesis in animal models, although they have also been shown to be cytotoxic *in vitro*. Chronic opioid use may trigger a switch in G protein-coupled mu opioid receptor signaling from AC inhibitory to stimulatory pathways resulting in increased barrier function and decreased permeability. Mu opioid receptor antagonists are used clinically in the treatment and management of opioid overdose and addiction, and also to counteract unwanted side effects in opioid analgesic regimes (Leppert 2010; Lobmaier et al. 2010). Unfortunately some mu opioid receptor antagonists such as naloxone and naltrexone, which are often used in the treatment for opioid overdose or addiction, can induce acute withdrawal symptoms (van Dorp et al. 2007). This has lead to the development of mu opioid receptor antagonists with limited bioavailability. Methylnaltrexone, due to its positive charge cannot pass through the blood–brain barrier and therefore does not affect analgesia or induce withdrawal, but does relieve the peripheral effects of opioids such as constipation and itching (Diego et al. 2009). The use of opioid antagonists to counter the effects of opioids on vascular barrier dysfunction is currently being investigated. A number of studies have shown that naltrexone and naloxone inhibit opioid-stimulated endothelial cell proliferation, angiogenesis and barrier permeability (Dai et al. 2008, 2010; Wen et al. 2011). Methylnaltrexone has also been shown to inhibit opiate induced increases in permeability and angiogenesis and potentiate the effects of other anti-angiogenic drugs *in vivo* (Mathew et al. 2011; Singleton et al. 2006b, 2007, 2010). Since opioids are widely used during the treatment of several classes of disease and injury, further research is needed to fully elucidate the contribution of both endogenous and clinically administered opiates in the regulation (and dysregulation) of endothelial barrier function. This understanding will aid in the development of novel therapeutics and treatment strategies for a wide range of vascular-related diseases.

## References


Abbott NJ, Patabendige AA, Dolman DE, Yusof SR, Begley DJ (2010) Structure and function of the blood–brain barrier. Neurobiol Dis 37:13–25

Afsharimani B, Cabot PJ, Parat MO (2011) Morphine use in cancer surgery. Front Pharmacol 2:46

Al-Hasani R, Bruchas MR (2011) Molecular mechanisms of opioid receptor-dependent signaling and behavior. Anesthesiology 115:1363–1381

Belcheva MM, Szucs M, Wang D, Sadee W, Coscia CJ (2001) Mu-Opioid receptor-mediated ERK activation involves calmodulin-dependent epidermal growth factor receptor transactivation. J Biol Chem 276:33847–33853

Birukova AA, Fu P, Xing J, Cokic I, Birukov KG (2010) Lung endothelial barrier protection by iloprost in the 2-hit models of ventilator-induced lung injury (VILI) involves inhibition of Rho signaling. Transl Res 155:44–54

Chang SL, Felix B, Jiang Y, Fiala M (2001) Actions of endotoxin and morphine. Adv Exp Med Biol 493:187–196

Curry FR, Adamson RH (2010) Vascular permeability modulation at the cell, microvessel, or whole organ level: towards closing gaps in our knowledge. Cardiovasc Res 87:218–229

Dai X, Cui SG, Wang T, Liu Q, Song HJ, Wang R (2008) Endogenous opioid peptides, endomorphin-1 and -2 and deltorphin I, stimulate angiogenesis in the CAM assay. Eur J Pharmacol 579: 269–275

Dai X, Song HJ, Cui SG, Wang T, Liu Q, Wang R (2010) The stimulative effects of endogenous opioids on endothelial cell proliferation, migration and angiogenesis *in vitro*. Eur J Pharmacol 628:42–50

Dejana E, Orsenigo F, Molendini C, Baluk P, McDonald DM (2009a) Organization and signaling of endothelial cell-to-cell junctions in various regions of the blood and lymphatic vascular trees. Cell Tissue Res 335:17–25

Dejana E, Tournier-Lasserve E, Weinstein BM (2009b) The control of vascular integrity by endothelial cell junctions: molecular basis and pathological implications. Dev Cell 16:209–221

Diego L, Atayee R, Helmons P, von Gunten CF (2009) Methylnaltrexone: a novel approach for the management of opioid-induced constipation in patients with advanced illness. Expert Rev Gastroenterol Hepatol 3:473–485

Donahoe RM, Vlahov D (1998) Opiates as potential cofactors in progression of HIV-1 infections to AIDS. J Neuroimmunol 83:77–87

Fujioka N, Nguyen J, Chen C, Li Y, Pasrija T, Niehans G, Johnson KN, Gupta V, Kratzke RA, Gupta K (2011) Morphine-induced epidermal growth factor pathway activation in non-small cell lung cancer. Anesth Analg 113:1353–1364

Gardner-Nix J (2002) Opioids causing peripheral edema. J Pain Symptom Manage 23:453–455

Gintzler AR, Chakrabarti S (2006) Post-opioid receptor adaptations to chronic morphine; altered functionality and associations of signaling molecules. Life Sci 79:717–722

Glattard E, Welters ID, Lavaux T, Muller AH, Laux A, Zhang D, Schmidt AR, Delalande F, Laventie BJ, Dirrig-Grosch S et al (2010) Endogenous morphine levels are increased in sepsis: a partial implication of neutrophils. PLoS One 5:e8791

Gupta K, Kshirsagar S, Chang L, Schwartz R, Law PY, Yee D, Hebbel RP (2002) Morphine stimulates angiogenesis by activating proangiogenic and survival-promoting signaling and promotes breast tumor growth. Cancer Res 62:4491–4498

Hawkins BT, Davis TP (2005) The blood–brain barrier/neurovascular unit in health and disease. Pharmacol Rev 57:173–185

Huet O, Dupic L, Harrois A, Duranteau J (2011) Oxidative stress and endothelial dysfunction during sepsis. Front Biosci 16:1986–1995
Koodie L, Ramakrishnan S, Roy S (2010) Morphine suppresses tumor angiogenesis through a HIF-1alpha/p38MAPK pathway. Am J Pathol 177:984–997
Lam CF, Chang PJ, Huang YS, Sung YH, Huang CC, Lin MW, Liu YC, Tsai YC (2008) Prolonged use of high-dose morphine impairs angiogenesis and mobilization of endothelial progenitor cells in mice. Anesth Analg 107:686–692
Le Guelte A, Dwyer J, Gavard J (2011) Jumping the barrier: VE-cadherin, VEGF and other angiogenic modifiers in cancer. Biol Cell 103:593–605
Lee WL, Liles WC (2011) Endothelial activation, dysfunction and permeability during severe infections. Curr Opin Hematol 18:191–196
Leo S, Nuydens R, Meert TF (2009) Opioid-induced proliferation of vascular endothelial cells. J Pain Res 2:59–66
Leppert W (2010) The role of opioid receptor antagonists in the treatment of opioid-induced constipation: a review. Adv Ther 27:714–730
Liu HC, Anday JK, House SD, Chang SL (2004) Dual effects of morphine on permeability and apoptosis of vascular endothelial cells: morphine potentiates lipopolysaccharide-induced permeability and apoptosis of vascular endothelial cells. J Neuroimmunol 146:13–21
Lobmaier P, Gossop M, Waal H, Bramness J (2010) The pharmacological treatment of opioid addiction – a clinical perspective. Eur J Clin Pharmacol 66:537–545
Mahajan SD, Aalinkeel R, Sykes DE, Reynolds JL, Bindukumar B, Fernandez SF, Chawda R, Shanahan TC, Schwartz SA (2008) Tight junction regulation by morphine and HIV-1 tat modulates blood–brain barrier permeability. J Clin Immunol 28:528–541
Martin TA, Jiang WG (2009) Loss of tight junction barrier function and its role in cancer metastasis. Biochim Biophys Acta 1788:872–891
Mathew B, Lennon FE, Siegler J, Mirzapoiazova T, Mambetsariev N, Sammani S, Gerhold LM, LaRiviere PJ, Chen CT, Garcia JG et al (2011) The novel role of the mu opioid receptor in lung cancer progression: a laboratory investigation. Anesth Analg 112:558–567
Miano JM, Berk BC (2006) HDAC7 supports vascular integrity. Nat Med 12:997–998
Milligan G (2005) Opioid receptors and their interacting proteins. Neuromolecular Med 7:51–59
Moore TM, Chetham PM, Kelly JJ, Stevens T (1998) Signal transduction and regulation of lung endothelial cell permeability: interaction between calcium and cAMP. Am J Physiol 275: L203–L222
Ocasio FM, Jiang Y, House SD, Chang SL (2004) Chronic morphine accelerates the progression of lipopolysaccharide-induced sepsis to septic shock. J Neuroimmunol 149:90–100
Paolinelli R, Corada M, Orsenigo F, Dejana E (2011) The molecular basis of the blood brain barrier differentiation and maintenance: is it still a mystery? Pharmacol Res 63:165–171
Puana R, McAllister RK, Hunter FA, Warden J, Childs EW (2008) Morphine attenuates microvascular hyperpermeability via a protein kinase A-dependent pathway. Anesth Analg 106:480–485
Ruan X, Tadia R, Couch JP, Ruan J, Chiravuri S (2008) Severe peripheral edema during an outpatient continuous epidural morphine infusion trial in a patient with failed back surgery syndrome. Pain Physician 11:363–367
Sacerdote P (2006) Opioids and the immune system. Palliat Med 20(suppl 1):s9–15
Schallmach E, Steiner D, Vogel Z (2006) Adenylyl cyclase type II activity is regulated by two different mechanisms: implications for acute and chronic opioid exposure. Neuropharmacology 50:998–1005
Sharma SK, Nirenberg M, Klee WA (1975) Morphine receptors as regulators of adenylate cyclase activity. Proc Natl Acad Sci U S A 72:590–594
Singleton PA, Moss J (2010) Effect of perioperative opioids on cancer recurrence: a hypothesis. Future Oncol 6:1237–1242
Singleton PA, Dudek SM, Chiang ET, Garcia JG (2005) Regulation of sphingosine 1-phosphate-induced endothelial cytoskeletal rearrangement and barrier enhancement by S1P1 receptor, PI3 kinase, Tiam1/Rac1, and alpha-actinin. Faseb J 19:1646–1656

Singleton PA, Dudek SM, Ma SF, Garcia JG (2006a) Transactivation of sphingosine 1-phosphate receptors is essential for vascular barrier regulation: novel role for hyaluronan and CD44 receptor family. J Biol Chem 281:34381–34393

Singleton PA, Lingen MW, Fekete MJ, Garcia JG, Moss J (2006b) Methylnaltrexone inhibits opiate and VEGF-induced angiogenesis: role of receptor transactivation. Microvasc Res 72:3–11

Singleton PA, Mambetsariev N, Lennon FE, Mathew B, Siegler JH, Moreno-Vinasco L, Salgia R, Moss J, Garcia JG (2010) Methylnaltrexone potentiates the anti-angiogenic effects of mTOR inhibitors. J Angiogenes Res 2:5

Singleton PA, Moreno-Vinasco L, Sammani S, Wanderling SL, Moss J, Garcia JG (2007) Attenuation of vascular permeability by methylnaltrexone: role of mOP-R and S1P3 transactivation. Am J Respir Cell Mol Biol 37:222–231

Skrupky LP, Kerby PW, Hotchkiss RS (2011) Advances in the management of sepsis and the understanding of key immunologic defects. Anesthesiology 115:1349–1362

Snyder GL, Greenberg S (2010) Effect of anaesthetic technique and other perioperative factors on cancer recurrence. Br J Anaesth 105:106–115

Surapisitchat J, Beavo JA (2011) Regulation of endothelial barrier function by cyclic nucleotides: the role of phosphodiesterases. Handb Exp Pharmacol 204:193–210

Tegeder I, Geisslinger G (2004) Opioids as modulators of cell death and survival – unraveling mechanisms and revealing new indications. Pharmacol Rev 56:351–369

Ustun F, Durmus-Altun G, Altaner S, Tuncbilek N, Uzal C, Berkarda S (2011) Evaluation of morphine effect on tumour angiogenesis in mouse breast tumour model, EATC. Med Oncol 28:1264–1272

van Dorp EL, Yassen A, Dahan A (2007) Naloxone treatment in opioid addiction: the risks and benefits. Expert Opin Drug Saf 6:125–132

Vandenbroucke E, Mehta D, Minshall R, Malik AB (2008) Regulation of endothelial junctional permeability. Ann N Y Acad Sci 1123:134–145

Waeber C, Blondeau N, Salomone S (2004) Vascular sphingosine-1-phosphate S1P1 and S1P3 receptors. Drug News Perspect 17:365–382

Waters C, Pyne S, Pyne NJ (2004) The role of G-protein coupled receptors and associated proteins in receptor tyrosine kinase signal transduction. Semin Cell Dev Biol 15:309–323

Wen H, Lu Y, Yao H, Buch S (2011) Morphine induces expression of platelet-derived growth factor in human brain microvascular endothelial cells: implication for vascular permeability. PLoS One 6:e21707

Yousif S, Saubamea B, Cisternino S, Marie-Claire C, Dauchy S, Scherrmann JM, Decleves X (2008) Effect of chronic exposure to morphine on the rat blood–brain barrier: focus on the P-glycoprotein. J Neurochem 107:647–657

Yuan SY, Rigor RR (2010) Regulation of endothelial barrier function. Morgan & Claypool Life Sciences, San Rafael

Zhang L, Zhao H, Qiu Y, Loh HH, Law PY (2009) Src phosphorylation of micro-receptor is responsible for the receptor switching from an inhibitory to a stimulatory signal. J Biol Chem 284:1990–2000

# Chapter 5
# Iatrogenic Angiogenesis

**Kalpna Gupta**

**Abstract** The medicinal powers of opium poppy-derived extracts now called 'opioids' and the importance of vasculature in maintaining life were realized by ancient civilizations. However, the association of the two with each other has emerged in the last decade. Opioid receptors, including the mu opioid receptor (MOR) which mediates opioid analgesia, are present on the endothelium. Analgesic opioids such as morphine and its congeners stimulate growth- and survival promoting signaling directly via MOR and also by co-activating receptor tyrosine kinases for vascular endothelial growth factor receptor 2, platelet-derived growth factor receptor β, etc. in the endothelial cells. Opioid signaling translates into increased tumor angiogenesis, tumor growth, metastases and reduced survival in mice. Additionally, opioids modulate the tumor microenvironment by acting on diverse cellular milieu of the tumor. Increased density of MOR in human tumors as compared to normal tissue, suggests a role for MOR in cancer. Based on experimental studies and MOR expression on human tumors it is critical to examine the role of opioids in cancer progression and survival in patients treated with opioids for severe pain.

**Keywords** Angiogenesis • Cancer • Endothelium • Metastases • Morphine • Opioid • Pain

## Abbreviations

| | |
|---|---|
| 11C-CFN | 11C-carfentanil |
| 11C-MeNTI | 11C-methylnaltrindole |

K. Gupta, Ph.D. (✉)
Department of Medicine, Division of Hematology, Oncology and Transplantation, Vascular Biology Center, University of Minnesota, Mayo Mail Code 480, 420 Delaware Street SE, Minneapolis, MN 55455, USA
e-mail: gupta014@umn.edu

M.-O. Parat (ed.), *Morphine and Metastasis*, DOI 10.1007/978-94-007-5678-6_5, 

| | |
|---|---|
| cAMP | cyclic adenosine monophosphate |
| COX | Cyclooxygenase |
| DOR | delta opioid receptor |
| GPCRs | G-coupled protein receptors |
| GRK | GPCR kinase |
| KOR | kappa opioid receptor |
| MNTX | methylnaltrexone |
| MAPK | mitogen-activated protein kinase |
| MOR | mu opioid receptor |
| NO | nitric oxide |
| NOS | NO synthase |
| NOP-R | nociceptin/Orphanin FQ receptor |
| NSCLC | non-small cell lung cancer |
| PDGF | platelet-derived growth factor |
| PDGFR-β | platelet-derived growth factor receptor-β |
| PET | Positron emission tomography |
| POMC | proopiomelanocortin |
| PGE2 | prostaglandin E2 |
| Akt | protein kinase B |
| RAVE | Relative activity versus endocytosis |
| STAT-3 | signal transducer and activator of transcription-3 |
| SCLC | small cell lung cancer |
| S1P3R | sphingosine-1 phosphate receptor |
| VEGF | vascular endothelial growth factor |
| VEGFR2, Flk1 | VEGF receptor-2 |

## 5.1 Introduction

Opioids, originating from opium poppy (*Papaver somniferum*), remain the most widely used analgesics to treat severe pain. However, their euphoria generating and healing power on one hand, and addiction and side effects on the other have turned them into a double-edged sword. Use of opium as a medicine was described in the 1700s. During the 1700s the term ‘angiogenesis’ also came into existence (Table 5.1). The first opioid receptor (OR; delta) was cloned in 1992, close to the discovery of vascular endothelial growth factor (VEGF), the endothelial cell-specific growth factor that promotes angiogenesis. Thus, the existence and development of opioids and angiogenesis followed parallel paths during history (Table 5.1). Once consumed either orally or injected into the body, opioids travel through the circulation to the target tissue, physically contacting the endothelial cells (ECs) lining the blood vessels. The presence of ORs was described on the endothelium soon after their discovery, thus arguing for the role of opioids in angiogenesis via opioid-endothelial interaction. Angiogenesis is the growth of new vessels from the pre-existing blood

Table 5.1 The parallel histories of opioids and angiogenesis

| Opioids | Angiogenesis |
|---|---|
| 1500s–1600s: Opium refined into modern day drugs | 1600s: Physicians discover that the heart pumps blood |
| 1757: Linnaeus classifies the opium poppy | 1787: John Hunter coins the term "angiogenesis" |
| Research on pain and nervous system effects ↓ | Research on endothelial cell activation/ inflammation ↓ |
| | 1971: Angiogenesis implicated in tumor metastasis |
| 1992: Delta Opioid Receptor cloned | |
| | 1989: VEGF discovered |
| → What is the role of opioids in angiogenesis? ← | |

History shows that both opioids and angiogenesis were considered of significant importance by thinkers, philosophers and scientists across the globe at about the same time. The realization of the significance of opioids in the process of angiogenesis is still in its infancy, despite the discovery of opioid receptors 2 decades ago

vessels, which plays a critical role in tumor progression and metastases. We provide an up to date review of the interaction of opioids with endothelium and their role in angiogenesis.

## 5.2 Classifications of Opioids and Their Receptors

On the basis of source of origin opioids may be classified as natural (derived from opiate alkaloid e.g. codeine and morphine), semi-synthetic (created by altering natural opioids e.g. oxycodone and hydrocodone), fully synthetic (synthesized in laboratories from non-opioid substances e.g. fentanyl, tramadol and methadone) or endogenous (naturally produced by body e.g. endorphin, enkephalins and dynorphin).

Based on molecular cloning and binding studies, four different classes of ORs are: mu-, delta- and kappa-OR (MOR, DOR and KOR, respectively) and nociceptin/ Orphanin FQ receptor (NOP-R). Each agonist is specific for a specific OR but can show cross-reactivity to other ORs with lower affinity. ORs are 7 transmembrane domain G-coupled protein receptors (GPCRs) coupled to pertussis toxin dependent Gi/Go type of G-proteins (Gupta et al. 2007). Upon receptor activation, both G-protein $\alpha$ and $\beta\gamma$ subunits interact with multiple effector systems, leading to the inhibition of adenyl cyclase and voltage-gated $Ca^{++}$ channels and stimulation of G-protein-activated inwardly rectifying $K^+$ channels. In contrast, chronic activation of OR may lead to the superactivation of adenyl cyclase and increased cyclic adenosine monophosphate (cAMP).

OR activity is similar to the classical GPCRs, where ligand binding initiates receptor phosphorylation by the GPCR kinase (GRK), followed by the recruitment of $\beta$-arrestin and uncoupling from the G-protein (Fig. 5.1). Uncoupled receptor is

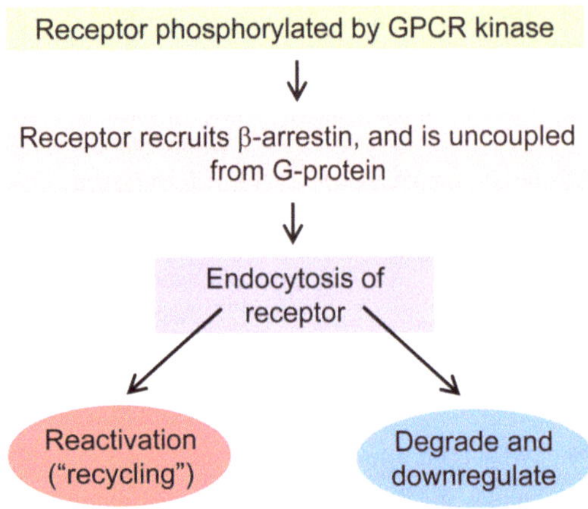


**Fig. 5.1** Opioid receptor regulation. Ligand binding to the opioid receptors induces phosphorylation of the GPCR by GPCR kinase. Phosphorylated receptor recruits β-arrestin, followed by uncoupling from the G-protein. The uncoupled receptor is then endocytosed and it is either recycled back (reactivation) or degraded (downregulation). In some instances the receptor remains phosphorylated and is not endocytosed. This is called receptor activation versus endocytosis (RAVE). Mu opioid receptor has a high RAVE value. Therefore, once activated by morphine it can remain activated for a prolonged time, thus amplifying the effect of morphine (Abbreviation: *GPCR* G-protein coupled receptor)

then endocytosed and re-activated or degraded (downregulated), depending upon the stimulus provided by the ligand binding and/or the property of the receptor. Importantly, MOR, the receptor that mediates the analgesic activity of morphine and its congeners, remains constitutively activated, even after the withdrawal of the ligand. When the receptor remains activated and does not get endocytosed the relative activity versus endocytosis (RAVE) is high. MOR has a high RAVE value, therefore, once morphine is added to the system it can lead to a prolonged activity of MOR.

## 5.3 Opioid Receptor Regulation

The expression of ORs is critical for the activity of endogenous and exogenous opioids, physiologically and in pathological conditions. Expression of ORs is modulated in a cell-specific manner by the cellular microenvironment constituted of pro-inflammatory cytokines and growth factors. For example, the pro-inflammatory cytokine IL-6 up regulates signal transducer and activator of transcription-3 (STAT-3) dependent MOR mRNA expression but not that of DOR in neuroblastoma cell line SH SY5Y cells (Borner et al. 2004). It is also contextual depending upon the cell type, pathology and organ system. For example in melanoma M2 cells lacking the actin cytoskeletal protein filamin A, morphine induced an upregulation of MOR, but not in the cells stably transfected with filamin A cDNA (Onoprishvili and Simon 2007).

On the other hand, nitric oxide (NO) upregulates MOR in intestinal inflammation in mice (Pol et al. 2005; Pol 2007). Since MOR stimulates NO production, the

NO-mediated up regulation of MOR suggests a feed-forward mechanism between NO and MOR. Similarly we observed that VEGF and serum induced MOR expression (Chen et al. 2006), while morphine up regulated VEGF receptor 2 (VEGFR2) expression in mouse retinal endothelial cells (Chen et al. 2006). VEGF-induces activation of VEGFR2 (Bartoli et al. 2003) via NO (Hood et al. 1998). Therefore, it is also possible that VEGFR2 activation leads to the stimulation of NO and subsequent upregulation of MOR. Increased NO and VEGFR2 are hallmarks of inflammation and cancer, and in-turn may lead to increased MOR expression in cancer (described below in detail).

## 5.4 Opioid Signaling in Endothelium

Morphine was shown to stimulate NO production in EC more than a decade ago (Fimiani et al. 1999; Prevot et al. 1998; Stefano et al. 1995, 1998). Morphine in the concentration of 1 μM and below 1 μM range stimulated NO release via MOR in human aortic endothelial cells and from rat aortic rings, leading to vasodilation (Stefano et al. 1995).

We found that a key mechanism of morphine-induced angiogenesis is NO-dependent mitogen-activated protein kinase (MAPK) and protein kinase B (Akt) phosphorylation (Gupta et al. 2002; Poonawala et al. 2005) (Fig. 5.2). Amongst the growth factors, VEGF is the only cytokine that stimulates MAPK phosphorylation and endothelial proliferation in a NO-dependent manner. Therefore, morphine acts like a growth factor in stimulating growth promoting signaling in endothelium. Importantly, morphine stimulated endothelial signaling, growth and survival at physiologically relevant doses in the μM range, but was cytotoxic in the mM range (Gupta et al. 2002). Table 5.2 shows different effects of morphine on signaling and function and the doses used.

Another key feature of angiogenesis and tumor growth is dysregulated expression of cyclin D1, leading to increased cell cycle progression and survival. Morphine at clinically relevant doses stimulates endothelial cyclin D1 and cell cycle progression and promotes survival by stimulating Akt phosphorylation (Gupta et al. 2002). Morphine stimulates angiogenic signaling in a manner similar to that VEGF-induced MAPK phosphorylation via NO. While morphine stimulates NO and MAPK phosphorylation directly, it also transactivates VEGF receptor, Flk1/VEGFR2 and platelet-derived growth factor receptor-β (PDGFR-β) via MOR on endothelial cells (Chen et al. 2006; Singleton et al. 2006).

MOR co-localized with CD31 positive tumor vasculature in human non-small cell lung cancer (NSCLC) biopsies, suggestive of upregulation of MOR and its association with increased tumor angiogenesis (Fujioka et al. 2011). Morphine and its congeners act as analgesics via MOR. Therefore, activation of MOR may have implications in promoting angiogenesis when morphine is used for analgesia.

In addition, MOR ligation by morphine and a MOR-specific agonist DAMGO leads to barrier dysfunction and increased permeability by activation of sphingosine-1 phosphate receptor (S1P3R) in human pulmonary microvascular endothelial cells

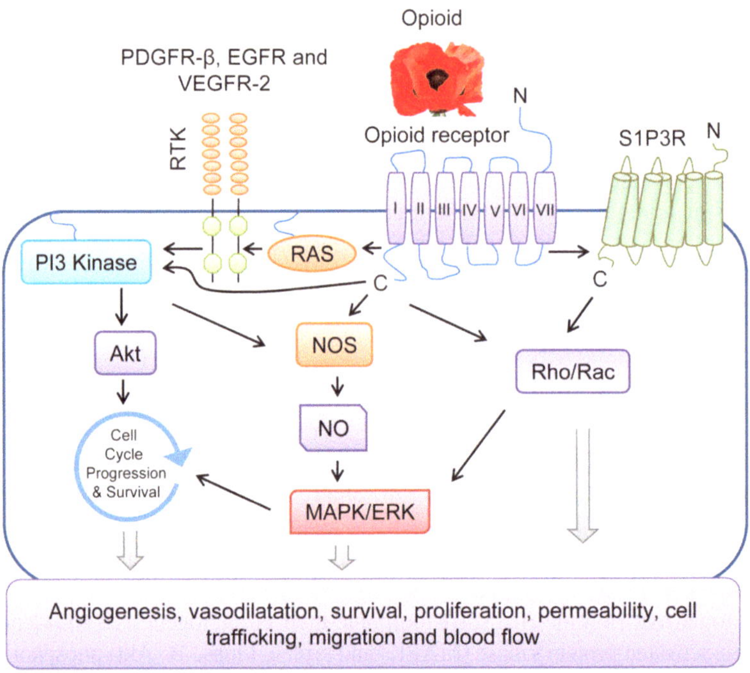


**Fig. 5.2** Opioid signaling in endothelium. Opioids stimulate growth- and survival-promoting signaling directly via their 7-transmembrane domain G-protein coupled receptors and/or by co-activating receptor tyrosine kinases for growth factors or other GPCRs (Abbreviations: *RTK* receptor tyrosine kinase, *S1P3R* sphingosine 1 phosphate receptor 3; *PI3 kinase* phosphoinositol 3 kinase; *NOS* nitric oxide synthase; *NO* nitric oxide; *MAPK/ERK* mitogen activated protein kinase/extracellular signal regulated kinase)

(Singleton et al. 2007). The MOR-specific antagonist methylnaltrexone (MNTX) inhibited the MOR-mediated barrier dysfunction, suggesting that MOR activation may play a critical role in endothelial physiology and angiogenesis. Peripheral MOR antagonists may be potentially useful in antagonizing the peripheral side effects of opioid analgesics.

Cyclooxygenase (COX), and production of its product prostaglandin E2 (PGE2) are stimulated by NO (Birnbaum et al. 2005; Nedelec et al. 2001; Salvemini et al. 1993, 1994). PGE2 is known to promote angiogenesis and tumor progression, and COX-2 inhibitors inhibit angiogenesis and tumor progression (Chang et al. 2004; Griffin et al. 2002; Leahy et al. 2002). Prostaglandins are involved in pain processing (Julius and Basbaum 2001; Malmberg and Yaksh 1992; Samad et al. 2001), and COX-2 inhibitors ameliorate the development of morphine tolerance (Wong et al. 2000). We observed that chronic morphine treatment at physiologically relevant doses leads to an upregulation of COX2 gene and protein expression and PGE2 in breast tumors in A/J mice (Farooqui et al. 2007). Furthermore chronic morphine treatment increased both inducible and endothelial NO synthase (NOS), hemoxygenase and COX-2 in mouse kidney (Arerangaiah et al. 2007; Weber et al. 2012).

**Table 5.2** Cellular effects of opioids

| Opioid | Dose | Cell type/system | Effect | Reference |
|---|---|---|---|---|
| Morphine | 0.01–100 μM | HDMEC | Cell proliferation and survival through NOS, MAPK/ERK, Akt signaling | Gupta et al. (2002) |
| Morphine | 0.75–1.0 mg/kg/day | SCK breast tumors in *A/J* mice | Stimulation of COX-2 signaling and increased PGE2 in tumors. Promotion of angiogenesis, tumor growth and metastases and reduced survival | Farooqui et al. (2007) |
| Morphine | 0.75–2 mg/kg/day | Peritoneal mast cells in mice | Degranulation, increase serotonin release, increase at inflammatory site | Manning et al. (2012) |
| Morphine | 10 nM | zebrafish | Regulate cell proliferation and neuronal differentiation via Wnt1 | Sanchez-Simon et al. (2012) |
| Morphine | 10–100 ng/ml | MCF7 and MDA-MB-231 human breast cancer cells | Increased migration by upregulating NET1 gene expression | Ecimovic et al. (2011) |
| Morphine | 0.714 mg/kg/day | Ehrlich ascites tumor cell xenograft in mice | Increased angiogenesis | Ustun et al. (2011) |
| Morphine | 0.01–10 μM | Human umbilical arterial endothelial cells | Increased cell proliferation via MAPK/ERK phosphorylation | Leo et al. (2009) |
| Morphine | 10–7 M | Human brain microvascular endothelial cells | Stimulation of PDGF-BB expression via MAPKs and Akt induced transcriptional activation of Egr-1; increased permeability | Wen et al. (2011) |
| Morphine | 10 μM | Lymphocytes | Cell survival through p53, Blc-2/Bax | Suzuki et al. (2003) |
| Morphine | 10 μM | mREC | Cell proliferation and survival through MAPK/ERK, Akt, STAT3 | Chen et al. (2006) |
| Morphine | 1–10 μM | HDMEC | Stimulates human microvascular endothelial cell proliferation and angiogenesis by activating MAPK/ERK phosphorylation via Gi/Go-coupled G protein receptors and nitric oxide | Gupta et al. (2002) |

(continued)

**Table 5.2** (continued)

| Opioid | Dose | Cell type/system | Effect | Reference |
|---|---|---|---|---|
| Morphine | 0.714 mg/kg mouse/day for first 15 days and then 1.43 mg/kg mouse/day | Human MCF7 breast cancer xenografts in nude mice | Angiogenesis and tumor progression | Gupta et al. (2002) |
| Morphine | 0.5 mg/kg/day to 1.5 mg/kg/day for 7 weeks | Transgenic mouse model of breast cancer, with rat C3(1) simian virus large tumor antigen. | Potentiates endothelial-pericyte interaction via PDGFR-β signaling. Promotion of tumor angiogenesis, and pericyte recruitment to the tumor vessels | Luk et al. (2012) |
| Morphine | 0.1–1 μM | HUVEC | PDGF-BB release and activation of PDGFR-b signaling | Luk et al. (2012) |
| Morphine | 10 μM | mREC | Promotes pro-angiogenic and survival-promoting signaling by stimulating MAPK/ERK and Akt phosphorylation in a time dependent manner like VEGF in mREC | Chen et al. (2006) |
| Morphine, fentanyl, hydromorphone | 1.5 mg/g, 5 μg/g, 0.2 mg/g base cream, respectively applied topically | Ischemic wounds in rats | Increased angiogenesis and acceleration of wound healing by upregulation of eNOS, iNOS, Flk1 | Poonawala et al. (2005) |
| Morphine, DAMGO | 0.01, 0.1 and 1 μM | Human pulmonary vein microvascular endothelial cells | Transactivation of sphingosine-1-phosphate receptor, S1P3 via mu opioid receptor and RhoA/ROCK mediated signaling and vascular permeability | Singleton et al. (2007) |
| Morphine, DAMGO | 0.01–1 μM | HDMEC and HPMVEC | MOR mediated transactivation of VEGF receptor 2 and endothelial proliferation and migration | Singleton et al. (2006) |
| Morphine, DAMGO | 1 nM | Lewis lung carcinoma cells | Cell proliferation | Mathew et al. (2011) |
| MOR | overexpression | H358 non-small cell lung cancer cells and xenografts in mice | Increased proliferation, migration, invasion via Akt signaling; and increased tumor growth | Lennon et al. (2012) |

| | | | | |
|---|---|---|---|---|
| Methylnaltrexone | 0.1 μM | HPMVEC | Blockade of morphine and DAMGO-induced disruption of barrier function | Singleton et al. (2007) |
| Methylnaltrexone | 10 mg/kg | Lungs of C57BL/6 J mice | Blockade of LPS-induced vascular leakage | Singleton et al. (2007) |
| Methylnaltrexone | 10 mg/kg/day for 2 weeks | Lewis lung carcinoma growth in mice. | Inhibition of tumor growth and metastases | Mathew et al. (2011) |
| DAMGO | 1 nM | Cyclin-dependent kinase 5 (CDK5) | Cell survival through Cyclin-dependent kinase 5 (CDK-5) | Yuen et al. (2004) |
| DAMGO | 50 μM | Cortical Neurons | Cell survival | Hou et al. (1996) |
| DAMGO | 1 μM | HDMEC | Cell proliferation | Gupta et al. (2002) |
| DPDPE | | | | |
| U50488H | | | | |

Abbreviations: *DAMGO* ([d-Ala(2), N-Me-Phe (4), Gly(5)-ol]enkaphalin), *DPDPE* D-Penicillamine2-D-Penicillamine5-Enkephalin, *U50488H* selective kappa-opioid receptor agonist, *HPMVEC* human pulmonary microvascular endothelial cells, *HDMEC* human dermal microvascular endothelial cells, *HUVEC* human umbilical vein endothelial cells, *HBMECs* human brain microvessel endothelial cells, *MAPK/ERK* mitogen-activated protein kinase/extracellular signal-regulated kinase, *VEGF* vascular endothelial growth factor, *mREC* mouse retinal endothelial cells, *STAT3* signal transducer and activator of transcription 3, *PDGF* platelet-derived growth factor, *PDGFR-b* PDGF receptor-b, *COX2* cyclooxygenase 2, *PGE2* prostaglandin E2

Morphine increased blood flow in the kidney of mice via a NO- and opioid receptor-mediated mechanism (Arerangaiah et al. 2007). These observations argue for a vasoregulatory role of morphine in addition to its growth- and survival-promoting effect.

## 5.5 Opioids and Opioid Receptors Modulate Tumor Microenvironment

The presence of endogenous opioids and opioid receptors in human cancers based on immunoreactivity and ligand binding studies, respectively was shown on human tumors more than two decades ago (Fichna and Janecka 2004). Molecular and modern imaging techniques have confirmed the increased presence of opioid receptors in cancerous tissue as compared to normal tissue in human cancers. An important question in this regard is why are the opioid receptors upregulated in cancer?

Opioid peptides are synthesized and released by immune cells including macrophages, polymorphonuclear leukocytes (PMNs), and lymphocytes in addition to their central origin (Sacerdote 2007; Stein et al. 2003). The proopiomelanocortin (POMC) gene expression is under the control of chemokines, cytokines and pathogens (Rittner et al. 2007; Westly et al. 1986). This increases the likelihood that increased POMC gene products such as endorphins in tumors may be due to the infiltration of tumors by immune cells and increased levels of pro-inflammatory cytokines and growth factors. Positron emission tomography (PET) scanning for the binding of DOR antagonist 11C-methylnaltrindole (11C-MeNTI) and MOR agonist 11C-carfentanil (11C-CFN) showed high density of MOR and DOR binding sites in the tumorous region as compared to normal lung tissue in lung cancer patients with small cell lung cancer (SCLC) and NSCLC of the squamous and adenocarcinoma cell type (Madar et al. 2007). Similarly, stronger MOR immunoreactivity was observed in parts of the tumor as compared to normal mucosa in human colon cancer (Nylund et al. 2008). More recent studies performed by our group and others have clearly demonstrated increased expression of MOR in a variety of human lung cancer biopsies (Fujioka et al. 2011; Mathew et al. 2011). We found that increased MOR expression co-localized with the tumor cells as well as the vascular endothelium in the tumor (Fujioka et al. 2011). Experimentally, human NSCLC H358 cells overexpressing MOR led to increased tumor growth and metastases when xenografted into mice as compared to cells transfected with vector control (Lennon et al. 2012). Thus, the tumor micro-environment provides a fertile ground for the upregulation of both endogenous opioids and opioid receptors and MOR promotes tumor growth and metastases by utilizing distinct signaling pathways.

Opioid receptors including MOR and opioid peptides permeate the entire biological system including inflammatory cells and the central nervous system. The interactions of morphine with a variety of cells promoting an inflammatory milieu are beginning to emerge (Fig. 5.3). Morphine stimulates endothelial signaling directly, but it may also modulate the tumor microenvironment by interacting with

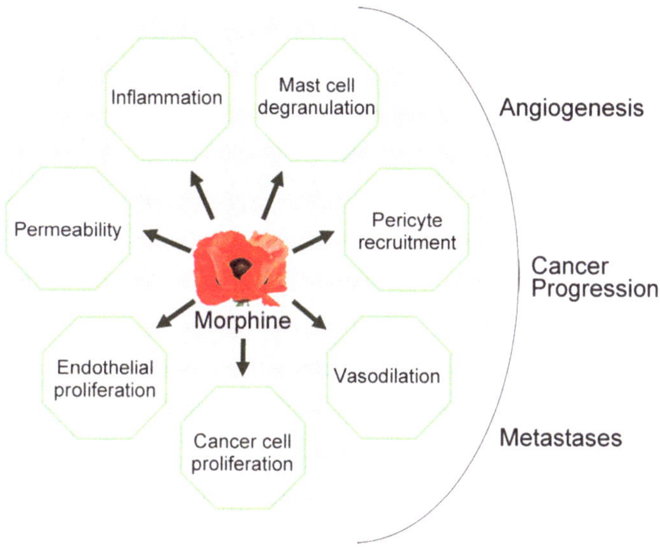


**Fig. 5.3** Opioids modulate tumor microenvironment. Opioids interact with multiple cell types within the tumor and in the circulation, which in turn modify the tumor microenvironment resulting in increased inflammation, mast cell degranulation, pericyte recruitment, permeability, proliferation and vasodilation. These cellular effects lead to enhancement of tumor angiogenesis, cancer progression and metastases

different cellular components in the tumor and by modulating the release of hormones from the pituitary-hypothalamus axis (Stephenson and Gupta 2006). We observed that morphine-induced COX-2 expression co-localized with the tumor cells, suggesting that morphine-induced COX-2 in tumors increases PGE2 release by cancer cells that stimulates tumor angiogenesis leading to tumor progression and reduced survival (Farooqui et al. 2007). The COX-2 inhibitor Celecoxib inhibited morphine-induced PGE2, angiogenesis and tumor progression and increased survival. Moreover, mice developed morphine tolerance that was also inhibited by COX-2, suggesting that COX2 upregulation may play a central role in the angiogenic activity and in developing tolerance to morphine. Identification and inhibition of such mechanisms that mediate critical components of cancer growth including angiogenesis, analgesia and cancer progression are essential to treat cancer pain effectively without promoting the disease.

Morphine also stimulates the expression of platelet-derived growth factor (PDGF)-BB in endothelial cells (Luk et al. 2012; Wen et al. 2011). Wen et al. found that morphine in physiologically relevant doses increased PDGF-BB expression in human brain microvascular endothelial cells and increased their permeability (Wen et al. 2011). Our laboratory showed increased release of PDGF-BB by morphine stimulation from human umbilical vein endothelial cells (Luk et al. 2012). In this study, morphine treatment of transgenic mice with breast cancer led to the co-activation of PDGFR-β on the pericytes and their recruitment to the tumor vasculature.

It is likely that morphine-induced PDGF-BB increases vascular permeability in the tumors. The recruitment of pericytes to the tumor vasculature may have implications in the promotion of tumor angiogenesis.

Mast cells are also considered important components of the tumor microenvironment which promote angiogenesis and tumor progression (Ribatti and Crivellato 2011). Using a functional assay employing amperometry we observed that morphine treatment of mice with chronic inflammation led to a significant increase in serotonin release suggestive of their increased degranulation (Manning et al. 2012). It is likely that morphine-induced mast cell degranulation contributes to increased angiogenesis and tumor progression.

Morphine also increases pro-inflammatory cytokines in the circulation and in tumors. Morphine increased tumor necrosis factor-α (TNF-α) significantly 12 h after administration when given during surgery (Gomez-Vazquez et al. 2012). Morphine also increases the release of several cytokines from microglial cells via MOR (Merighi et al. 2012). We observed that transgenic mice with breast cancer had elevated pro-inflammatory cytokines when treated with morphine for a few weeks as compared to those treated with PBS (unpublished observations). It is likely that morphine-induced angiogenesis, tumor progression and metastases observed in rodents are an outcome of its direct effects on tumor endothelium and that of the microenvironment that favors growth and survival of endothelial and tumor cells.

## 5.6 Relevance of Opioid-Induced Angiogenesis to Cancer Progression and Metastases

We and others have demonstrated that morphine stimulates angiogenesis in vitro and in vivo (Farooqui et al. 2007; Fujioka et al. 2011; Gupta et al. 2002; Lennon, et al. 2012; Luk et al. 2012; Mathew et al. 2011; Poonawala et al. 2005; Singleton et al. 2006, 2007). Morphine induced angiogenesis in human MCF-7 breast cancers in nude mice, in syngeneic mouse SCK breast cancer in A/J mice and in large T-antigen expressing spontaneously growing breast cancer in FVBN mice. Similarly morphine also promoted angiogenesis, cancer progression and metastases in Lewis lung cancer xenografts in mice (Mathew et al. 2011). Overexpression of MOR in H358 human lung cancer xenografts in mice led to increased tumor growth and metastases, suggesting that MOR activity contributes to cancer progression (Lennon et al. 2012). Therefore, it is likely that increased MOR expression reported for lung and colon cancer may have a role in cancer progression.

A human study shows an indirect increase in the recurrence of metastasis after opioid analgesia using morphine with general anesthesia as compared to paravertebral anesthesia (Exadaktylos et al. 2006). In this retrospective study the dose of morphine was not recorded, but it was used with general anesthesia post-operatively. The follow-up time was $32 \pm 5$ months after surgery. Furthermore, in spite of morphine use pain scores were higher in the general anesthesia group as compared to paravertebral anesthesia group. It is likely that increased recurrence in the general anesthesia group could be due to the cancer-promoting effect of morphine.

Experimental studies in rodents using clinically used doses of morphine unequivocally demonstrate the promotion of angiogenesis by morphine and MOR. Therefore, it is critical to evaluate the effect of morphine and its congeners on cancer progression in human studies and devise strategies to prevent the inadvertent effect of opioids on cancer without compromising analgesia.

**Acknowledgements** We thank Mihir Gupta and Hemant Kumar for assistance with figures and Ms Carol Taubert for the artwork and word processing. This work was funded by NIH grants, RO1 HL68802, HL103773, and CA109582.

## References

Arerangaiah R, Chalasani N, Udager AM, Weber ML, Manivel JC, Griffin RJ, Song CW, Gupta K (2007) Opioids induce renal abnormalities in tumor-bearing mice. Nephron Exp Nephrol 105:e80–89. doi:10.1159/000098564

Bartoli M, Platt D, Lemtalsi T, Gu X, Brooks SE, Marrero MB, Caldwell RB (2003) VEGF differentially activates STAT3 in microvascular endothelial cells. FASEB J 17:1562–1564. doi:10.1096/fj.02-1084fje

Birnbaum Y, Ye Y, Rosanio S, Tavackoli S, Hu ZY, Schwarz ER, Uretsky BF (2005) Prostaglandins mediate the cardioprotective effects of atorvastatin against ischemia-reperfusion injury. Cardiovasc Res 65:345–355. doi:10.1016/j.cardiores.2004.10.018

Borner C, Kraus J, Schroder H, Ammer H, Hollt V (2004) Transcriptional regulation of the human mu-opioid receptor gene by interleukin-6. Mol Pharmacol 66:1719–1726. doi:10.1124/mol.104.003806

Chang SH, Liu CH, Conway R, Han DK, Nithipatikom K, Trifan OC, Lane TF, Hla T (2004) Role of prostaglandin e2-dependent angiogenic switch in cyclooxygenase 2-induced breast cancer progression. Proc Natl Acad Sci U S A 101:591–596. doi:10.1073/pnas.2535911100

Chen C, Farooqui M, Gupta K (2006) Morphine stimulates vascular endothelial growth factor-like signaling in mouse retinal endothelial cells. Curr Neurovasc Res 3:171–180

Ecimovic P, Murray D, Doran P, McDonald J, Lambert DG, Buggy DJ (2011) Direct effect of morphine on breast cancer cell function in vitro: role of the net1 gene. Br J Anaesth 107:916–923. doi:10.1093/bja/aer259

Exadaktylos AK, Buggy DJ, Moriarty DC, Mascha E, Sessler DI (2006) Can anesthetic technique for primary breast cancer surgery affect recurrence or metastasis? Anesthesiology 105:660–664

Farooqui M, Li Y, Rogers T, Poonawala T, Griffin RJ, Song CW, Gupta K (2007) COX-2 inhibitor celecoxib prevents chronic morphine-induced promotion of angiogenesis, tumour growth, metastasis and mortality, without compromising analgesia. Br J Cancer 97:1523–1531. doi:10.1038/sj.bjc.6604057

Fichna J, Janecka A (2004) Opioid peptides in cancer. Cancer Metastasis Rev 23:351–366. doi:10.1023/B:CANC.0000031773.46458.63

Fimiani C, Mattocks D, Cavani F, Salzet M, Deutsch DG, Pryor S, Bilfinger TV, Stefano GB (1999) Morphine and anandamide stimulate intracellular calcium transients in human arterial endothelial cells: coupling to nitric oxide release. Cell Signal 11:189–193

Fujioka N, Nguyen J, Chen C, Li Y, Pasrija T, Niehans G, Johnson KN, Gupta V, Kratzke RA, Gupta K (2011) Morphine-induced epidermal growth factor pathway activation in non-small cell lung cancer. Anesth Analg 113:1353–1364. doi:ANE.0b013e318232b35a [pii] 10.1213/ANE.0b013e318232b35a

Gomez-Vazquez ME, Hernandez-Salazar E, Novelo-Otanez JD, Cabrera-Pivaral CE, Davalos-Rodriguez IP, Salazar-Paramo M (2012) Effect of endovenous morphine vs. ketorolac on proinflammatory cytokines during postoperative analgesia in laparoscopic cholecystectomy. Cir Cir 80:56–62

Griffin RJ, Williams BW, Wild R, Cherrington JM, Park H, Song CW (2002) Simultaneous inhibition of the receptor kinase activity of vascular endothelial, fibroblast, and platelet-derived growth factors suppresses tumor growth and enhances tumor radiation response. Cancer Res 62:1702–1706

Gupta K, Kshirsagar S, Chang L, Schwartz R, Law PY, Yee D, Hebbel RP (2002) Morphine stimulates angiogenesis by activating proangiogenic and survival-promoting signaling and promotes breast tumor growth. Cancer Res 62:4491–4498

Gupta M, Yunfang L, Gupta K (2007) Opioids as promoters and regulators of angiogenesis. In: Maragoudakis ME, Papadimitriou E (eds) Angiogenesis: basic science and clinical applications. Transworld Research Network, Kerala, pp 303–317

Hood JD, Meininger CJ, Ziche M, Granger HJ (1998) VEGF upregulates ecNOS message, protein, and NO production in human endothelial cells. Am J Physiol 274:H1054–H1058

Hou YN, Vlaskovska M, Cebers G, Kasakov L, Liljequist S, Terenius L (1996) A mu-receptor opioid agonist induces AP-1 and NF-kappa B transcription factor activity in primary cultures of rat cortical neurons. Neurosci Lett 212:159–162

Julius D, Basbaum AI (2001) Molecular mechanisms of nociception. Nature 413:203–210. doi:10.1038/35093019

Leahy KM, Ornberg RL, Wang Y, Zweifel BS, Koki AT, Masferrer JL (2002) Cyclooxygenase-2 inhibition by celecoxib reduces proliferation and induces apoptosis in angiogenic endothelial cells in vivo. Cancer Res 62:625–631

Lennon FE, Mirzapoiazova T, Mambetsariev B, Salgia R, Moss J, Singleton PA (2012) Overexpression of the mu-opioid receptor in human non-small cell lung cancer promotes akt and mtor activation, tumor growth, and metastasis. Anesthesiology. doi:10.1097/ALN.0b013e31824babe2

Leo S, Nuydens R, Meert TF (2009) Opioid-induced proliferation of vascular endothelial cells. J Pain Res 2:59–66

Luk K, Boatman S, Johnson KN, Dudek OA, Ristau N, Vang D, Nguyen J, Gupta K (2012) Influence of morphine on pericyte-endothelial interaction: implications for antiangiogenic therapy. J Oncol 2012:458385. doi:10.1155/2012/458385

Madar I, Bencherif B, Lever J, Heitmiller RF, Yang SC, Brock M, Brahmer J, Ravert H, Dannals R, Frost JJ (2007) Imaging delta- and mu-opioid receptors by pet in lung carcinoma patients. J Nucl Med 48:207–213

Malmberg AB, Yaksh TL (1992) Hyperalgesia mediated by spinal glutamate or substance p receptor blocked by spinal cyclooxygenase inhibition. Science 257:1276–1279

Manning BM, Hebbel RP, Gupta K, Haynes CL (2012) Carbon-fiber microelectrode amperometry reveals sickle-cell-induced inflammation and chronic morphine effects on single mast cells. ACS Chem Biol 7:543–551. doi:10.1021/cb200347q

Mathew B, Lennon FE, Siegler J, Mirzapoiazova T, Mambetsariev N, Sammani S, Gerhold LM, LaRiviere PJ, Chen CT, Garcia JG, Salgia R, Moss J, Singleton PA (2011) The novel role of the mu opioid receptor in lung cancer progression: a laboratory investigation. Anesth Analg 112:558–567. doi:ANE.0b013e31820568af [pii] 10.1213/ANE.0b013e31820568af

Merighi S, Gessi S, Varani K, Fazzi D, Mirandola P, Borea PA (2012) Cannabinoid CB(2) receptor attenuates morphine-induced inflammatory responses in activated microglial cells. Br J Pharmacol 166:2371–2385. doi:10.1111/j.1476-5381.2012.01948.x

Nedelec E, Abid A, Cipolletta C, Presle N, Terlain B, Netter P, Jouzeau J (2001) Stimulation of cyclooxygenase-2-activity by nitric oxide-derived species in rat chondrocyte: lack of contribution to loss of cartilage anabolism. Biochem Pharmacol 61:965–978

Nylund G, Pettersson A, Bengtsson C, Khorram-Manesh A, Nordgren S, Delbro DS (2008) Functional expression of mu-opioid receptors in the human colon cancer cell line, HT-29, and their localization in human colon. Dig Dis Sci 53:461–466. doi:10.1007/s10620-007-9897-y

Onoprishvili I, Simon EJ (2007) Chronic morphine treatment up-regulates mu opioid receptor binding in cells lacking filamin A. Brain Res 1177:9–18. doi:10.1016/j.brainres.2007.08.020

Pol O (2007) The involvement of the nitric oxide in the effects and expression of opioid receptors during peripheral inflammation. Curr Med Chem 14:1945–1955

Pol O, Sasaki M, Jimenez N, Dawson VL, Dawson TM, Puig MM (2005) The involvement of nitric oxide in the enhanced expression of mu-opioid receptors during intestinal inflammation in mice. Br J Pharmacol 145:758–766. doi:10.1038/sj.bjp. 0706227

Poonawala T, Levay-Young BK, Hebbel RP, Gupta K (2005) Opioids heal ischemic wounds in the rat. Wound Repair Regen 13:165–174. doi:10.1111/j.1067-1927.2005.130207.x

Prevot V, Rialas CM, Croix D, Salzet M, Dupouy JP, Poulain P, Beauvillain JC, Stefano GB (1998) Morphine and anandamide coupling to nitric oxide stimulates GnRH and CRF release from rat median eminence: neurovascular regulation. Brain Res 790:236–244

Ribatti D, Crivellato E (2011) Mast cells, angiogenesis and cancer. In: Gilfillan AM, Metcalfe DD (eds). Mast Cell Biology: contemporary and emerging topics. Landes Bioscience and Springer Science + Business Media, Austin, pp 270–288

Rittner HL, Labuz D, Richter JF, Brack A, Schafer M, Stein C, Mousa SA (2007) CXCR1/2 ligands induce p38 MAPK-dependent translocation and release of opioid peptides from primary granules in vitro and in vivo. Brain Behav Immun 21:1021–1032. doi:10.1016/j.bbi.2007.05.002

Sacerdote P (2007) Immune cell-derived opioid peptides: back to the future. Brain Behav Immun 21:1019–1020. doi:10.1016/j.bbi.2007.06.006

Salvemini D, Misko TP, Masferrer JL, Seibert K, Currie MG, Needleman P (1993) Nitric oxide activates cyclooxygenase enzymes. Proc Natl Acad Sci U S A 90:7240–7244

Salvemini D, Seibert K, Masferrer JL, Misko TP, Currie MG, Needleman P (1994) Endogenous nitric oxide enhances prostaglandin production in a model of renal inflammation. J Clin Invest 93:1940–1947. doi:10.1172/JCI117185

Samad TA, Moore KA, Sapirstein A, Billet S, Allchorne A, Poole S, Bonventre JV, Woolf CJ (2001) Interleukin-1beta-mediated induction of Cox-2 in the CNS contributes to inflammatory pain hypersensitivity. Nature 410:471–475. doi:10.1038/35068566

Sanchez-Simon FM, Ledo AS, Arevalo R, Rodriguez RE (2012) New insights into opioid regulatory pathways: influence of opioids on Wnt1 expression in zebrafish embryos. Neuroscience 200:237–247. doi:10.1016/j.neuroscience.2011.10.026

Singleton PA, Lingen MW, Fekete MJ, Garcia JG, Moss J (2006) Methylnaltrexone inhibits opiate and VEGF-induced angiogenesis: role of receptor transactivation. Microvasc Res 72:3–11. doi:10.1016/j.mvr.2006.04.004

Singleton PA, Moreno-Vinasco L, Sammani S, Wanderling SL, Moss J, Garcia JG (2007) Attenuation of vascular permeability by methylnaltrexone: role of mOP-R and S1P3 transactivation. Am J Respir Cell Mol Biol 37:222–231. doi:10.1165/rcmb.2006-0327OC

Stefano GB, Hartman A, Bilfinger TV, Magazine HI, Liu Y, Casares F, Goligorsky MS (1995) Presence of the mu3 opiate receptor in endothelial cells: coupling to nitric oxide production and vasodilation. J Biol Chem 270:30290–30293

Stefano GB, Salzet M, Magazine HI, Bilfinger TV (1998) Antagonism of LPS and IFN-gamma induction of iNOS in human saphenous vein endothelium by morphine and anandamide by nitric oxide inhibition of adenylate cyclase. J Cardiovasc Pharmacol 31:813–820

Stein C, Schafer M, Machelska H (2003) Attacking pain at its source: new perspectives on opioids. Nat Med 9:1003–1008. doi:10.1038/nm908

Stephenson EJ, Gupta K (2006) Existence and modus operandii of opioid receptors in endothelium. In: Aird W (ed) The endothelium: a comprehensive reference. Cambridge University Press, Cambridge, MA, pp 451–460

Suzuki S, Chuang LF, Doi RH, Chuang RY (2003) Morphine suppresses lymphocyte apoptosis by blocking p53-mediated death signaling. Biochem Biophys Res Commun 308:802–808

Ustun F, Durmus-Altun G, Altaner S, Tuncbilek N, Uzal C, Berkarda S (2011) Evaluation of morphine effect on tumour angiogenesis in mouse breast tumour model, EATC. Med Oncol 28:1264–1272. doi:10.1007/s12032-010-9573-5

Weber ML, Vang D, Velho PE, Gupta P, Crosson JT, Hebbel RP, Gupta K (2012) Morphine promotes renal pathology in sickle mice. Int J Nephrol Renovasc Dis 5:109–118

Wen H, Lu Y, Yao H, Buch S (2011) Morphine induces expression of platelet-derived growth factor in human brain microvascular endothelial cells: implication for vascular permeability. PLoS One 6:e21707. doi:10.1371/journal.pone.0021707

Westly HJ, Kleiss AJ, Kelley KW, Wong PK, Yuen PH (1986) Newcastle disease virus-infected splenocytes express the proopiomelanocortin gene. J Exp Med 163:1589–1594

Wong CS, Hsu MM, Chou R, Chou YY, Tung CS (2000) Intrathecal cyclooxygenase inhibitor administration attenuates morphine antinociceptive tolerance in rats. Br J Anaesth 85:747–751

Yuen JW, So IY, Kam AY, Wong YH (2004) Regulation of STAT3 by mu-opioid receptors in human neuroblastoma SH-SY5Y cells. Neuroreport 15:1431–1435

# Chapter 6
# Could Opioids Affect Cancer Recurrence or Metastases? Current Experimental and Translational Evidence

**Hilary Shanahan, Marie-Odile Parat, and Donal Buggy**

**Abstract** 'Firstly, do no harm' – a fundamental principle in the practice of medicine. Opioids have long been the mainstay in the treatment of acute and chronic cancer pain, but can opioids administered to cancer patients during the course of their treatment actually do more harm than good? This chapter examines the current experimental and translational research relating to opioids and their potential effect on cancer recurrence and metastases.

**Keywords** Opioids • Cancer recurrence • Metastases • Anaesthesia • Analgesia • Morphine • Pain

## Abbreviations

| | |
|---|---|
| BAEC | bovine aortic endothelial cells |
| JNK | c-Jun N-terminal kinase |
| COX-2 | cyclooxygenase-2 |
| CTL | cytotoxic T lymphocytes |

H. Shanahan • *D. Buggy (✉)
Department of Anaesthesia, Mater Misericordiae University Hospital, Dublin 7, Ireland

*Outcomes Research Consortium, Cleveland Clinic, Cleveland, OH, USA
e-mail: donal.buggy@ucd.ie

M.-O. Parat
School of Pharmacy, Pharmacy Australia Centre of Excellence, University of Queensland, 20 Cornwall Street, Woolloongabba, Brisbane, QLD 4102, Australia

Outcomes Research Consortium, Cleveland Clinic, Cleveland, OH, USA
e-mail: m.parat@uq.edu.au

M.-O. Parat (ed.), *Morphine and Metastasis*, DOI 10.1007/978-94-007-5678-6_6, 

| | |
|---|---|
| DNA | deoxyribo nucleic acid |
| ERAS | enhanced recovery after surgery |
| FADD | Fas-associated death domain |
| HPA | hypothalamic-pituitary-adrenal |
| IL-10 | interleukin 10 |
| IL-1β | interleukin 1β |
| IL-2 | interleukin 2 |
| JNK | c-Jun N-terminal Kinase |
| LLC | Lewis Lung Carcinoma |
| MSC | mesenchymal stem cell |
| MMP | matrix metalloproteinase |
| MAPK | mitogen-activated protein kinase |
| MOR | mu opioid receptor |
| NK | Natural killer |
| NSCLC | non small cell lung cancer |
| NFκB | nuclear factor kappa B |
| PDGFR-β | PDGF receptor-beta |
| PDGF-BB | platelet-derived growth factor-BB |
| PGE2 | prostaglandin E2 |
| ROS | reactive oxygen species |
| TGF-β | transforming growth factor beta |
| TNFα | tumour necrosis factor alpha |
| uPA | urokinase type plasminogen activator |
| VEGF | vascular endothelial growth factor |

## 6.1 Introduction

This chapter outlines the most recent, relevant state of knowledge on the influence of opioid drugs on cancer cell biology and outcomes. Because clinical evidence is currently limited, the work summarized here pertains to experimental models of cancer, including cell and tissue culture and live animal models.

The balance between cancer cell proliferation and apoptosis, and the ability of those surviving cells to invade other tissues and migrate to distant host sites influence the impact of cancer on a patient. Opioids have been shown to directly affect cancer cell proliferation, apoptosis, invasion, and migration and have also been shown to indirectly influence cancer spread via effects on the immune system, angiogenesis and local inflammation. However reports in the literature are conflicting as to whether opioids ultimately facilitate or hinder cancer cell survival and spread, and this chapter outlines the current evidence.

## 6.2 Direct Effects of Opioids on Cancer Cells

### *6.2.1 Direct Effect of Opioids on Cancer Cell Proliferation and Apoptosis*

A number of receptor types and mechanisms of action have been proposed as playing a role in cancer cell proliferation. Opioid receptors, which are present not only in the central and peripheral nervous system, but in cancer cells (Maneckjee and Minna 1990, Hatzoglou et al. 1996, Kampa et al. 1997, Fichna et al. 2005, Nylund et al. 2008, Kerros et al. 2009, Mathew et al. 2011), play an important role in the effect of endogenous and exogenous opioids on cancer cells. A number of studies in the 1990s have shown a decrease in tumor cell proliferation following the administration of morphine, by activation of cancer cell opioid receptors (Maneckjee and Minna 1990, Maneckjee et al. 1990, Kampa et al. 1997). It has also been proposed that interaction with the somatostatin receptor SSTR2 (Hatzoglou et al. 1995), inhibition of nuclear factor kappa B (NFκB) activation (Sueoka et al. 1998), suppression of tumour necrosis alpha (TNFα) expression (Sueoka et al. 1996) and p53 activation (Tegeder et al. 2003) have a role to play in decreasing tumor cell proliferation following administration of morphine. More recent studies however have yielded conflicting results. Mathew et al. found a 5–10 fold increase in mu opioid receptor (MOR) expression in lung samples of patients with non small cell lung cancer (NSCLC) and in several NSCLC cell lines, and in contrast to the studies conducted in the 1990s found an increase in proliferation of Lewis lung cancer cells when exposed to morphine in vitro, an effect thought to involve the mu opioid receptor. This effect was attenuated by the MOR antagonist, methylnaltrexone, suggesting mu opioid receptors as a potential target in lung cancer therapy (Mathew et al. 2011).

While most of the evidence suggests an inhibition of proliferation of tumor cells when exposed to morphine, there are conflicting studies which show an increase in tumor cell proliferation (Mathew et al. 2011) as discussed, or indeed no change to proliferation (Nylund et al. 2008, Gach et al. 2009) when cancer cells are exposed to morphine. The diversity in cancer cell lines studied and the differing concentrations in morphine used could explain this conflicting evidence in relation to cancer cell proliferation.

Apoptosis of cancer cells is also directly affected by opioid administration. A number of studies have found an increase in apoptosis when cancer cells were exposed to morphine (Maneckjee and Minna 1994, Zagon and McLaughlin 2003, Tegeder et al. 2003, Yin et al. 2006, Lin et al. 2009). Maneckjee and Minna examined the relationship of opioids and nicotine to lung cancer cell apoptosis. They found that opioids induced while nicotine suppressed apoptosis. There was a dose dependent increase in DNA fragmentation, characteristic of apoptosis, 2 h post opioid administration. The apoptosis associated with opioids appeared to be suppressed by nicotine, supporting other literature suggesting nicotine is a cancer-promoting agent (Maneckjee and Minna 1994). A reduction in protein kinase C activity appeared to be involved in morphine associated apoptosis. Tegeder et al. proposed a naloxone-independent p53 stabilization, and subsequent increase in pro-apoptotic factors p21, Bax, Fas death receptor, as the mechanism of action involved in the increased apoptosis of cancer cells observed at higher concentrations of morphine (≥500 μm) (Tegeder et al. 2003). Zagon and McLaughlin studied three human cancer cell lines, HT-29 colon adenocarcinoma, MIA PaCa-2 pancreatic adenocarcinoma, and CAL-27 head and neck squamous cell carcinoma, and found a pro-apoptotic effect of morphine partially reversed by naloxone (Zagon and McLaughlin 2003). Human Jurkat leukaemia cells were investigated by Yin et al. and the authors observed an increase in apoptosis when cells were exposed to morphine, possibly via activation of Fas-associated death domain (FADD)/p53, anti-apoptotic PI3 Kinase/Akt and NF-kB pathways (Yin et al. 2006). The effects of chronic high doses of morphine on neuroblastoma cells were investigated by Lin et al. and they noted that there was a dose-dependent increase in cell apoptosis. Activation of c-Jun N-terminal kinase (JNK) by morphine led to an increase in reactive oxygen species (ROS), up-regulation of pro-apoptotic protein Bim and down-regulation of anti-apoptotic protein Bcl-2, leading to an increase in cytochrome c release and capase-3 and -9 activation (Lin et al. 2009).

Hatsukari et al. hypothesized that many previous studies found a pro-apoptotic effect of morphine because a cytotoxic dose rather than a clinically relevant dose of morphine was used ($10^{-8}$ M was considered a clinically relevant concentration). They found that millimolar concentrations of morphine showed higher cytotoxicity against human tumor cell lines than against normal human cells. At a clinically used concentration of morphine, early apoptotic markers were seen in two cancer cell lines, HL-60 and A549, and higher numbers of necrotic cells in MCF7 cancer cells. The clinical concentration of morphine failed to activate any caspase species and induced only trace amounts of DNA fragmentation, in contrast to cytotoxic concentrations of morphine (Hatsukari et al. 2007). However most recently Qin et al. showed that concentrations of morphine as low as 0.1 μM induced caspase-9 and -3 expression, decreased survivin and NFκB expression, and caused cell cycle arrest in G2/M (Qin et al. 2012).

In contrast to the above studies which show the pro-apoptotic effect of morphine, Lin et al. found that morphine inhibited the anti-tumour activity of doxorubin in neuroblastoma cells in a dose-dependent manner. Inhibition of reactive oxygen species and cytochrome c release by morphine, and inhibition of NFκB activation, was proposed as a mechanism for inhibition of doxorubin-induced apoptosis when neuroblastoma cells were exposed to morphine (Lin et al. 2007).

### *6.2.2 Direct Effects of Opioids on Invasion and Migration of Cancer Cells*

There is also conflicting evidence in relation to opioids role in cancer cell invasion, extravasation, migration and growth in a secondary tissue. Administration of morphine was shown to increase breast adenocarcinoma cell migration in vitro, and this effect was mediated by increased expression of the NET1 gene (Ecimovic et al. 2011). In a different study, mu opioid receptors were implicated as important mediators of lung cancer progression. The authors found that over-expression of the MOR in human non-small cell lung cancer promotes Akt and mTOR activation, tumor growth, extravasation and migration (Lennon et al. 2012).

Nylund et al. found that morphine at a concentration of 0.1 μM markedly increased secretion of urokinase type plasminogen activator (uPA), a protease involved in invasion and metastases of cancer cells (Nylund et al. 2008). The effect of mu opioid agonists on uPA was also investigated by Gach et al., who showed that morphine greatly stimulated uPA secretion in the MCF-7 breast cancer cell line (Gach et al. 2009). Epidermal growth factor pathway activation by morphine via opioid receptors has also been implicated in human NSCLC cell invasion (Fujioka et al. 2011).

In contrast, some studies have found that opioids inhibit cancer cell invasion and migration, or have no effect. The effect of morphine on matrix metalloproteinase (MMP)-2 and -9, proteolytic enzymes which are involved in the degradation of the extracellular matrix and cancer cell invasion, was examined in the breast cancer cell line MCF-7. Opioids seemed to inhibit MMP secretion, and this inhibition was not reversed by the opioid receptor antagonist naloxone. The authors proposed that the nitric oxide system mediated the effect of morphine (Gach et al. 2011). Harimaya et al. examined the behavior of colon 26-L5 cancer cells when exposed to morphine and found that morphine significantly reduced the number of tumor colonies and lung metastases, by inhibition of adhesion and migration of the colon cancer cells to extracellular matrix and invasion through basement membrane (Harimaya et al. 2002). On the other hand, Zagon et al. studied the effects of opioid agonists and antagonists on seven cancer cell lines of three types of human cancers; pancreatic, colon and squamous cell carcinoma of the head and neck. They found that there was no effect on cancer cell migration, chemotaxis or invasion of any cancer cell line (Zagon et al. 2007).

## 6.3 Indirect Effects of Opioids

### *6.3.1 Effects of Opioids on Angiogenesis*

Angiogenesis or the formation of new blood vessels, is important for tumor growth and spread, and there is conflicting evidence regarding the effect of opioids on tumor angiogenesis. There are a number of in vitro tissue/cell studies, and in vivo animal studies investigating the effect of morphine on angiogenesis. Leo et al. evaluated the effects of morphine on endothelial cells, which are known to play an important role in angiogenesis. They found that, in vitro, morphine stimulates the proliferation of endothelial cells – known to express the μ3 opioid receptor – thus potentially promoting angiogenesis. This effect of morphine was proposed to involve the MAPK pathway (Leo et al. 2009). Singleton et al. examined the in vitro effect of morphine on human dermal microvascular endothelial cells. They unveiled that morphine increased their proliferation and migration via vascular endothelial growth factor receptor transactivation (Singleton et al. 2006). The effect of morphine on mouse retinal endothelial cells in vitro was examined by Chen et al. who found an increase in proliferation and survival of endothelial cells via a mitogen-activated protein kinase (MAPK) pathway (Chen et al. 2006). There are a number of live animal studies that show an increase in tumor angiogenesis upon exposure to opioids. Ustun et al. conducted a preclinical study, and found that there was increased angiogenesis in mouse breast cancers when animals were exposed to analgesic doses of morphine (equivalent to 50 mg per day for a 70 kg human). Morphine-triggered angiogenesis is this study was demonstrated by microvessel density and Doppler sonography (Ustun et al. 2011). In another mouse study, Luk et al. 2012, found that clinically relevant doses of morphine stimulated tumor angiogenesis, increased pericyte recruitment and coverage of tumor vessels in mice breast cancers by potentiation of endothelial-pericyte interaction. Furthermore, morphine stimulated platelet-derived growth factor-BB (PDGF-BB) secretion from endothelial cells and PDGF receptor-beta (PDGFR-β) signaling in pericytes in vitro (Luk et al. 2012). Gupta et al. showed earlier that morphine stimulates human microvascular endothelial cell proliferation and angiogenesis by activating pro-angiogenic signaling, and promotes breast tumor growth in a human breast tumor xenograft model in mice, at a clinically relevant concentration (Gupta et al. 2002). In contrast to these studies, Koodie et al. found that morphine administered at clinically relevant doses significantly suppressed tumor cell-induced angiogenesis using Lewis lung carcinoma cells (LLCs) in mice. They showed that morphine significantly reduced blood vessel density, vessel branching, and vessel length when compared with placebo treatment and that this effect was abolished in mice co-administered with the opioid receptor antagonist, naltrexone, and in mu-opioid receptor knockout mice, demonstrating the involvement of the opioid receptors in vivo. The authors suggested that suppression of the hypoxia-induced mitochondrial p38 MAPK pathway mediated the inhibitory effect of morphine on angiogenesis (Koodie et al. 2010).

### *6.3.2 Effects on Opioids on Immune Function*

The immune system plays an important role in cancer cell proliferation/apoptosis and spread. Tumor cells express antigens which attract attack from the cells of the immune system; activated T cells, natural killer cells and cytokines. Opioids may have an effect on the cellular immune response by acting on cells of the immune system directly, or by modulating the hypothalamic-pituitary-adrenal (HPA) axis response to pain or a surgical stimulus. In a live mouse study that was designed to assess the effect of morphine on Herpes Simplex Virus reactivation, Mojadadi et al. found that acute morphine administration led to a decrease in cytolytic T lymphocyte activity and lymphocyte proliferation (Mojadadi et al. 2009). In contrast, Fuggetta et al. examined, in vitro, the effect of morphine on the generation of human cytotoxic T lymphocytes (CTL) and found that morphine at graded concentrations enhanced CTL responses by directly affecting the induction phase of T-dependent cell-mediated immunity, but did not affect natural killer (NK) cell activity (Fuggetta et al. 2005). Different opioids exert differing effects on the immune system. Franchi et al. conducted an in vivo study of rats and looked at immune responses to a surgical stimulus, immunosupressive properties of different opioids, and the ability of those opioids to attenuate the immune response to surgery. They found that a surgical stimulus in itself decreased NK cell function and increased tumour metastases. They also found that both morphine and fentanyl were immunosupressive in themselves, even in the absence of a surgical stimulus. However buprenorphine, a potent partial mu-agonist, was found to attenuate the effect of a surgical stimulus on the HPA axis and prevent the increase in tumor metastasis caused by a surgical stimulus (Franchi et al. 2007). Shavit et al. also looked at the immunosupressive properties of fentanyl in a live animal study in the absence of concomitant surgical stress. They concluded that fentanyl suppressed natural killer cell cytotoxicity, and increased the risk of tumor metastasis (Shavit et al. 2004). In an in vitro human peripheral blood lymphocyte study, Ohara et al. suggested that there was no induction of apoptotic processes by morphine (Ohara et al. 2005). In contrast, in a live rat model, tramadol was found to be protective by suppressing the effect of surgery on NK cell function and metastatic diffusion of NK-sensitive MADB106 tumor cells to the lung. Morphine, in contrast, did not attenuate surgery-induced increase in lung metastasis in that study. Not only did tramadol prevent surgery-induced NK suppression but in non-operated rats tramadol actually increased NK activity (Gaspani et al. 2002). Forget et al. studied the effects of fentanyl on NK function at different time points after a surgical stimulus in a live animal study. Fentanyl was administered 1 h before a laparotomy and the activity of natural killer cells was quantified in vitro at different time points up to 8 days post administration. There was a rapid increase in NK activity in the first 24 h post operatively which was then followed by a significant decrease in NK function which eventually returned to baseline level at 8 days post operatively. Fentanyl suppressed NK function with or without surgery (Forget et al. 2010a).

### *6.3.3 Effects of Opioids on Inflammation*

Local inflammation appears to play a role in cancer cell proliferation. In a retrospective study of women who underwent mastectomy and axillary clearance for breast cancer treatment Forget et al. found that intraoperative use of the non-steroidal anti-inflammatory drug ketorolac decreased the risk of cancer relapse in breast cancer patients when compared to other analgesics (Forget et al. 2010b). Farooqui et al. showed that 2 weeks of chronic morphine administration at clinically relevant doses stimulated pro-inflammatory cyclooxygenase-2 (COX-2) and prostaglandin E2 (PGE2) production in a breast cancer model in mice. Administration of the

COX-2 inhibitor celecoxib was found to prevent this morphine-induced stimulation of COX-2 and PGE2 production, and subsequently reduced angiogenesis, tumour growth, metastasis and mortality (Farooqui et al. 2007).

### *6.3.4 Indirect Promigratory Effect of Morphine Demonstrated Ex Vivo*

We have tested the effect of in vivo administered morphine in a bioresponse assay. Mice were injected intraperitoneally with 10 mg/kg morphine sulfate every 12 h for 3 consecutive days, and their serum, collected on the fourth day, was used to test cell migration in a modified Boyden chamber assay towards control medium or medium added with 2 % serum prepared from morphine and saline-treated mice. The serum from morphine-treated mice was a much more potent chemoattractant than the serum of saline-treated mice (Fig. 6.1a). This was seen both with bovine aortic endothelial cells (BAEC) (proangiogenic effect) and 4T1 breast cancer cells (prometastatic effect), although the difference seemed more dramatic in the 4T1 migration assay than in the BAEC migration assay. The blood samples were taken 12 h after the last injection of morphine, and we verified that this effect was not mediated by residual morphine in the serum of morphine-treated mice using both ELISA- and mass spectrometry-based methods. Furthermore, the increased cell migration induced by serum from morphine-treated mice was not reversed by naloxone (Fig. 6.1b), confirming that the pro-migratory effect of serum from morphine-treated mice is not due to the presence of residual morphine at the time of blood collection. Lastly, we demonstrated that the soluble factor(s) present in the serum from morphine-treated mice is (are) sensitive to heat inactivation by comparing the migration of 4T1 breast cancer cells to morphine- and saline-treated mouse serum that had been heat-inactivated or left unheated. Control cells migrated towards serum-free medium. This experiment (Fig. 6.1c) showed that the difference in pro-migratory capability between serum from morphine- and saline-treated mice was abrogated by heat inactivation ($p<0.001$). Taken together, our results indicate that an indirect effect of morphine treatment on cell migration is observed. This indirect effect may come from heat-sensitive, soluble factor(s) present in serum after pharmacologically active concentrations of morphine have been eliminated from the circulation. Similar bioresponse approaches have been employed in the setting of clinical studies (Deegan et al. 2009, 2010).

**Fig. 6.1** (continued) Control cells migrated towards serum-free medium (random migration). Error bars represent SEM. $n=4$ mice per group. $^{**}p<0.01$, $^{***}p<0.001$. (**b**) Migration of 4 T1 cells was induced by placing 2% serum from morphine treated mice in the bottom wells of the migration chamber. Some serum samples were added with naloxone 0.07 μM to neutralize the potential residual morphine present in the serum. Error bars represent SEM. $n=3$ mice. (**c**) Serum from morphine or saline-treated mice was heat-inactivated at 56°C for 1 h. Migration of 4T1 cells was induced by placing 2% heat inactivated serum or unheated serum in the bottom wells of the migration chamber. Control cells migrated towards serum-free medium (random migration). Error bars represent SEM. $n=8$ wells per sample

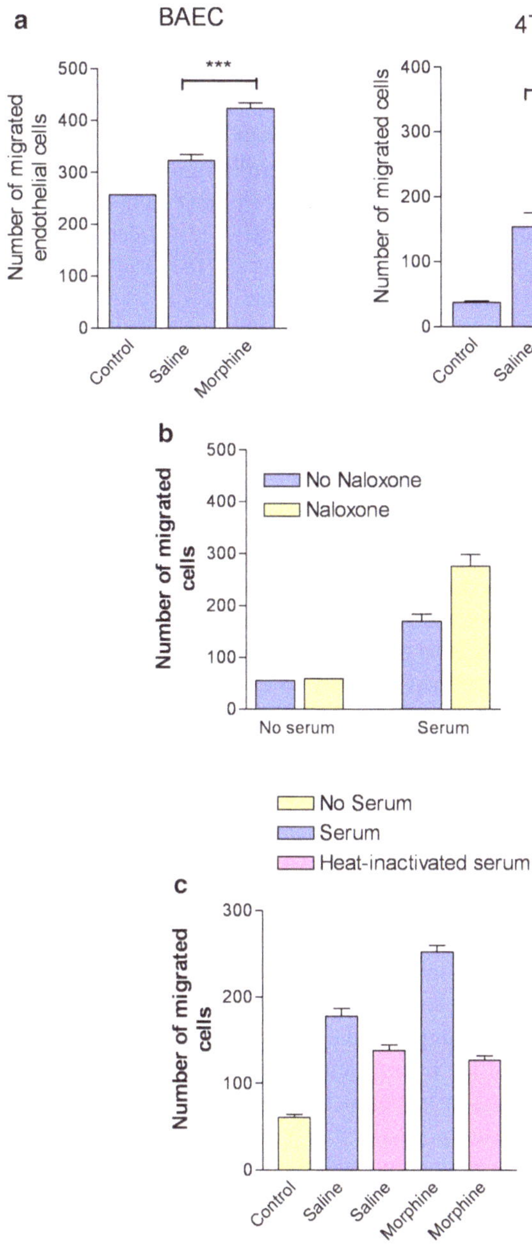


**Fig. 6.1** Ex vivo promigratory effects of morphine. To test the effect of in vivo administered morphine in a bioresponse assay, mice were injected intraperitoneally with 10 mg/kg morphine sulfate every 12 h for 3 consecutive days. Control mice were injected with 0.9 % NaCl. All mice within one experiment were littermates. Twelve hours after the last injection, the mice were euthanized for blood collection and the serum samples were used as chemoattractant in a modified Boyden chamber assay. All experiments were approved by institutional animal ethics committee. (**a**) Bovine aortic endothelial cells (BAEC) and 4T1 breast cancer cells were induced to migrate towards 2% serum isolated from littermates that had been treated for 3 consecutive days with morphine or saline.

## 6.4 Clinical Trials on Opioid Versus Non Opioid Analgesia for Cancer Surgery

There is evidence that suggests that it is pain itself, and its effects on the sympathetic and immune system, that stimulate cancer proliferation and spread, and that the control of pain, by any method, is paramount in preventing cancer metastasis and recurrence. Macfarlane et al. prospectively followed patients who complained of pain (widespread and regional pain) over 8 years and found an interesting association between reporting of widespread pain and death from cancer in the medium and longterm (Macfarlane et al. 2001). Smith et al. also found that implantable intrathecal drug delivery systems that lead to better pain control in refractory cancer pain also lead to an improved survival for those patients (Smith et al. 2002). Supporting the hypothesis that control of pain in itself is beneficial to patients is the success of the enhanced recovery after surgery (ERAS) pathway, which aims to reduce the stress response to surgery. This has been shown to reduce length of stay and complications for patients after major colorectal surgery (Varadhan et al. 2010). Furthermore Sasamura et al. found that pain control, by either morphine administration or neurectomy of the sciatic nerve reduced tumor growth and lung metastasis in mice inoculated with painful tumours in the hind paw (Sasamura et al. 2002).

Is there however one method of analgesia for cancer surgery that confers benefits to a patient over another method? Many studies have been designed to evaluate the effects of opioid versus regional analgesia on cancer proliferation and spread. It is hypothesized that as regional anaesthesia reduces opioid requirements and regional lympathic flow during surgery, its use may be associated with benefits for the cancer patient (Ismail et al. 2010). Deegan et al. exposed cells of the estrogen receptor-negative MDA-MB-231 breast cancer cell line to the serum of breast cancer surgery patients who either received anaesthesia with the inhalational agent sevoflurane and opioid analgesia, or to anaesthesia with a propofol infusion and paravertebral analgesia. There was inhibition of proliferation, but not migration, of breast cancer cells in vitro to a greater extent in the propofol/paravertebral anaesthesia/analgesia serum group than in the sevoflurane/opioid serum group (Deegan et al. 2009). Looney et al. conducted a randomised controlled clinical trial looking at the effect of anaesthetic technique for breast cancer surgery on factors thought to promote angiogenesis and metastasis in breast cancer, vascular endothelial growth factor (VEGF)-C and transforming growth factor beta (TGF-β). They also compared propofol/paravertebral and sevoflurane/opioid anaesthetic techniques. They found that patients randomised to the propofol/paravertebral group had less pain at 2 h postoperatively than the sevoflurane/opioid group. Post-operative VEGF C serum levels were increased in the sevoflurane/opioid group but unchanged in the propofol/regional group. In contrast, TGF-β levels were decreased post operatively in the sevoflurane/opioid group. The authors concluded that anaesthetic technique alters the concentration of factors in the serum associated with angiogenesis in breast cancer (Looney et al. 2010). Deegan et al. further tested the effect of analgesia techniques in breast cancer surgery (propofol/paravertebral group versus sevoflurane/

opioid group), and their effects on circulating levels of protumorigenic cytokines, antitumorigenic cytokines and matrix metalloproteinases (MMPs). They found that in patients with propofol/paravertebral anesthesia-analgesia there was a greater percentage decrease in postoperative compared with preoperative interleukin 1β (IL-1β), a significant attenuation in elevated MMP-3 and MMP-9, and a significant increase in interleukin 10 (IL-10) compared with patients in the sevoflurane/opioid group (Deegan et al. 2010).

There are also a number of studies researching the effect of the anaesthesia/analgesia technique on cancer outcome. Biki et al. retrospectively reviewed the medical records of patients who underwent open radical prostatectomy for invasive prostate cancer, and compared post-operative prostate-specific antigen (PSA) values in patients who received opioid analgesia or epidural analgesia. PSA was used as a biochemical marker of cancer recurrence. They found that epidural analgesia was associated with significantly less risk of biochemical cancer recurrence than opioid analgesia (Biki et al. 2008). However, in a similar study where the authors looked at disease recurrence after radical prostatectomy and compared groups that received general anaesthesia alone versus general/regional anaesthesia, no difference was observed between the groups in terms of disease free survival (Tsui et al. 2010). Wuethrich et al. compared opioid/ketorolac analgesia to thoracic epidural analgesia for retropubic radical prostatectomy in a retrospective analysis study and found that epidural analgesia was associated with a reduced risk of cancer progression but there was no significant difference between the two techniques in biochemical recurrence-free survival, cancer specific survival, or overall survival (Wuethric et al. 2010). Forget et al. conducted a retrospective analysis of cancer recurrence in patients who underwent retropubic radical prostatectomies, and found that sufentanil administration was associated with an increased risk of cancer recurrence, whereas epidural analgesia which used a combination of local anaesthetic and opioid was not associated with an effect on cancer recurrence (Forget et al. 2011).

Studies investigating other types of cancer have been performed. De Oliveira et al. investigated the time to tumor recurrence in patients who underwent surgery for ovarian cancer, and found that the use of epidural analgesia was associated with a longer cancer recurrence-free time (De Oliveira et al. 2011). Cummings et al. looked retrospectively at a large cohort of patients who underwent surgery for non-metastatic colorectal cancer and found that epidural analgesia was associated with a survival benefit, but their study did not prove an association between epidural use and decreased cancer recurrence (Cummings et al. 2012). A retrospective analysis of colorectal cancer patients who underwent surgery was undertaken by Day et al. Patients received either regional or opioid analgesia and the authors found that there was no significant difference between the groups in overall or disease-free survival (Day et al. 2012). Exadaktylos et al. studied retrospective data on breast cancer patients undergoing mastectomy and axillary clearance and compared perioperative paravertebral analgesia and opioid analgesia. The authors suggested that there was a reduced risk of cancer recurrence or metastasis associated with the paravertebral analgesia (Exadaktylos et al. 2006). Lucchinetti et al. investigated the local anaesthetics lidocaine, ropivacaine, and bupivacaine, and their effect on mesenchymal

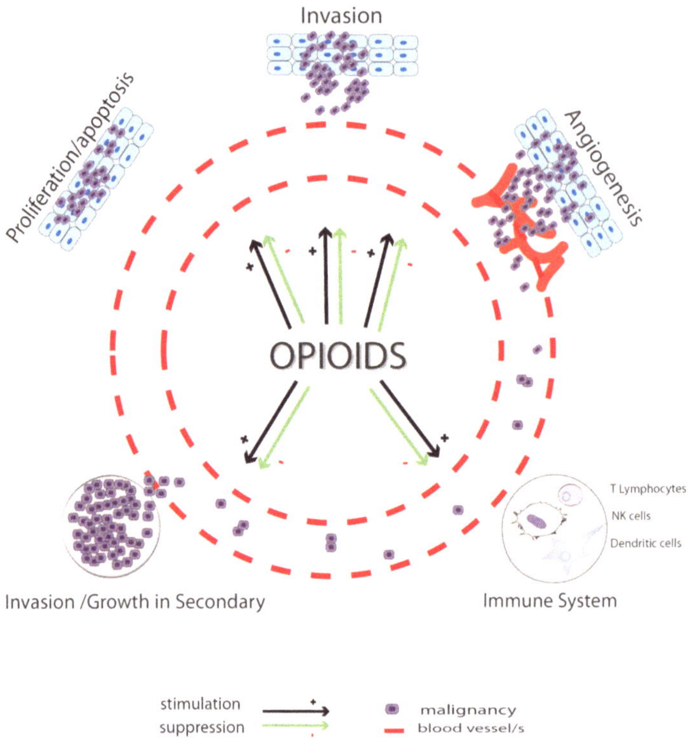


**Fig. 6.2** stages of cancer cell proliferation and spread, and conflicting evidence in relation to the effect of opioids on each stage

stem cell (MSC) biology. All local anaesthetics significantly reduced MSC proliferation which has implications for tumor growth and spread as well as wound healing after surgery (Lucchinetti et al. 2012). Finally, a prospective large muticentre randomised control trial comparing general anaesthesia for major abdominal cancer surgery, with or without the use of perioperative epidural analgesia unveiled that use of epidural was not associated with improved cancer-free survival in this group of patients (Myles et al. 2011).

## 6.5 Evidence for Acute Versus Chronic Opioid Use

Opioids are used for both acute pain management in cancer surgery and the treatment of chronic cancer pain. The effect of opioids on responses involved in cancer growth and metastasis may be different in the cancer surgery perioperative setting and in cancer patients with chronic pain. For example, in a preclinical study Martucci et al. have compared the effect of acute fentanyl and buprenorphine administration to longer term use on the immune system of mice. Parameters studied were lymphoproliferation, natural killer cell activity and interleukin 2 (IL-2) and interferon gamma production. Buprenorphine was shown to have little effect on the immune system at any time, and fentanyl was immunosuppressive in the short term but this became less relevant with a longer duration of use, with return of immune system to baseline after 7 days of continuous fentanyl administration (Martucci et al. 2004).

## 6.6 Conclusion

Opioids have long been the mainstay of pain therapy in cancer patients in both the acute perioperative period and in the treatment of refractory pain in cancer, but could they be causing more harm than good? As demonstrated, there is conflicting evidence as to the effect of opioid administration on every aspect of cancer cell biology (Fig. 6.2), and clinical studies evaluating opioid versus non opioid analgesia for cancer surgery are also conflicting and overall non-conclusive. Is it reasonable to use alternatives to opioids where possible before these questions have been answered? Or is it more important to treat pain aggressively in these patients and attenuate the stress response where possible? Large prospective muticentre randomised control trials are needed to answer many important questions in this area.

**Acknowledgements** We thank JoAnne Baran and Linda Gricourt for technical help.

## References

Biki B, Mascha E, Moriarty DC, Fitzpatrick JM, Sessler DI, Buggy DJ (2008) Anesthetic technique for radical prostatectomy surgery affects cancer recurrence: a retrospective analysis. Anesthesiology 109:180–187

Chen C, Farooqui M, Gupta K (2006) Morphine stimulates vascular endothelial growth factor-like signaling in mouse retinal endothelial cells. Curr Neurovasc Res 3:171–180

Cummings KC III, Xu F, Cummings LC, Cooper GS (2012) A comparison of epidural analgesia and traditional pain management effects on survival and cancer recurrence after colectomy: a population-based study. Anesthesiology 116:797–806

Day A, Smith R, Jourdan I, Fawcett W, Scott M, Rockall T (2012) Retrospective analysis of the effect of postoperative analgesia on survival in patients after laparoscopic resection of colorectal cancer. Br J Anaesth 109:185–190

De Oliveira G Jr, Ahmad S, Schink JC, Singh DK, Fitzgerald PC, McCarthy RJ (2011) Intraoperative neuraxial anesthesia but not postoperative neuraxial analgesia is associated with increased relapse-free survival in ovarian cancer patients after primary cytoreductive surgery. Reg Anesth Pain Med 36:271–277

Deegan CA, Murray D, Doran P, Ecimovic P, Moriarty DC, Buggy DJ (2009) Effect of anaesthetic technique on oestrogen receptor-negative breast cancer cell function in vitro. Br J Anaesth 103:685–690

Deegan CA, Murray D, Doran P, Moriarty DC, Sessler DI, Mascha E, Kavanagh BP, Buggy DJ (2010) Anesthetic technique and the cytokine and matrix metalloproteinase response to primary breast cancer surgery. Reg Anesth Pain Med 35:490–495

Ecimovic P, Murray D, Doran P, McDonald J, Lambert DG, Buggy DJ (2011) Direct effect of morphine on breast cancer cell function in vitro: role of the NET1 gene. Br J Anaesth 107:916–923
Exadaktylos AK, Buggy DJ, Moriarty DC, Mascha E, Sessler DI (2006) Can anesthetic technique for primary breast cancer surgery affect recurrence or metastasis? Anesthesiology 105:660–664
Farooqui M, Li Y, Rogers T, Poonawala T, Griffin RJ, Song CW, Gupta K (2007) COX-2 inhibitor celecoxib prevents chronic morphine-induced promotion of angiogenesis, tumour growth, metastasis and mortality, without compromising analgesia. Br J Cancer 97:1523–1531
Fichna J, Krajewska U, Rozalski M, Mirowski M, Janecka A (2005) Characterization of the [125I] endomorphin-2 binding sites in the MCF7 breast cancer cell line. Peptides 26:295–299
Forget P, Collet V, Lavand'homme P, De Kock M (2010a) Does analgesia and condition influence immunity after surgery? Effects of fentanyl, ketamine and clonidine on natural killer activity at different ages. Eur J Anaesthesiol 27:233–240
Forget P, Vandenhende J, Berliere M, Machiels JP, Nussbaum B, Legrand C, De Kock M (2010b) Do intraoperative analgesics influence breast cancer recurrence after mastectomy? A retrospective analysis. Anesth Analg 110:1630–1635
Forget P, Tombal B, Scholtes JL, Nzimbala J, Meulders C, Legrand C, Van Cangh P, Cosyns JP, De Kock M (2011) Do intraoperative analgesics influence oncological outcomes after radical prostatectomy for prostate cancer? Eur J Anaesthesiol 28:830–835
Franchi S, Panerai AE, Sacerdote P (2007) Buprenorphine ameliorates the effect of surgery on hypothalamus-pituitary-adrenal axis, natural killer cell activity and metastatic colonization in rats in comparison with morphine or fentanyl treatment. Brain Behav Immun 21:767–774
Fuggetta MP, Di Francesco P, Falchetti R, Cottarelli A, Rossi L, Tricarico M, Lanzilli G (2005) Effect of morphine on cell-mediated immune responses of human lymphocytes against allogeneic malignant cells. J Exp Clin Cancer Res 24:255–263
Fujioka N, Nguyen J, Chen C, Li Y, Pasrija T, Niehans G, Johnson KN, Gupta V, Kratzke RA, Gupta K (2011) Morphine-induced epidermal growth factor pathway activation in non small cell lung cancer. Anesth Analg 113:1353–1364
Gach K, Szemraj J, Fichna J, Piestrzeniewicz M, Delbro DS, Janecka A (2009) The influence of opioids on urokinase plasminogen activator on protein and mRNA level in MCF-7 breast cancer cell line. Chem Biol Drug Des 74:390–396
Gach K, Szemraj J, Wyrebska A, Janecka A (2011) The influence of opioids on matrix metalloproteinase-2 and -9 secretion and mRNA levels in MCF-7 breast cancer cell line. Mol Biol Rep 38:1231–1236
Gaspani L, Bianchi M, Limiroli E, Panerai AE, Sacerdote P (2002) The analgesic drug tramadol prevents the effect of surgery on natural killer cell activity and metastatic colonization in rats. J Neuroimmunol 129:18–24
Gupta K, Kshirsagar S, Chang L, Schwartz R, Law PY, Yee D, Hebbel RP (2002) Morphine stimulates angiogenesis by activating proangiogenic and survival-promoting signaling and promotes breast tumor growth. Cancer Res 62:4491–4498
Harimaya Y, Koizumi K, Andoh T, Nojima H, Kuraishi Y, Saiki I (2002) Potential ability of morphine to inhibit the adhesion, invasion and metastasis of metastatic colon 26-L5 carcinoma cells. Cancer Lett 187:121–127
Hatsukari I, Hitosugi N, Ohno R, Hashimoto K, Nakamura S, Satoh K, Nagasaka H, Matsumoto I, Sakagami H (2007) Induction of apoptosis by morphine in human tumor cell lines in vitro. Anticancer Res 27:857–864
Hatzoglou A, Ouafik L, Bakogeorgou E, Thermos K, Castanas E (1995) Morphine cross-reacts with somatostatin receptor SSTR2 in the T47D human breast cancer cell line and decreases cell growth. Cancer Res 55:5632–5636
Hatzoglou A, Bakogeorgou E, Castanas E (1996) The antiproliferative effect of opioid receptor agonists on the T47D human breast cancer cell line, is partially mediated through opioid receptors. Eur J Pharmacol 296:199–207
Ismail H, Ho KM, Narayan K, Kondalsamy-Chennakesavan S (2010) Effect of neuraxial anaesthesia on tumour progression in cervical cancer patients treated with brachytherapy: a retrospective cohort study. Br J Anaesth 105:145–149

Kampa M, Bakogeorgou E, Hatzoglou A, Damianaki A, Martin PM, Castanas E (1997) Opioid alkaloids and casomorphin peptides decrease the proliferation of prostatic cancer cell lines (LNCaP, PC3 and DU145) through a partial interaction with opioid receptors. Eur J Pharmacol 335:255–265

Kerros C, Cavey T, Sola B, Jauzac P, Allouche S (2009) Somatostatin and opioid receptors do not regulate proliferation or apoptosis of the human multiple myeloma U266 cells. J Exp Clin Cancer Res 28:77

Koodie L, Ramakrishnan S, Roy S (2010) Morphine suppresses tumor angiogenesis through a HIF-1alpha/p38MAPK pathway. Am J Pathol 177:984–997

Lennon FE, Mirzapoiazova T, Mambetsariev B, Salgia R, Moss J, Singleton PA (2012) Overexpression of the mu-opioid receptor in human non-small cell lung cancer promotes Akt and mTOR activation, tumor growth, and metastasis. Anesthesiology 116:857–867

Leo S, Nuydens R, Meert TF (2009) Opioid-induced proliferation of vascular endothelial cells. J Pain Res 2:59–66

Lin X, Li Q, Wang YJ, Ju YW, Chi ZQ, Wang MW, Liu JG (2007) Morphine inhibits doxorubicin-induced reactive oxygen species generation and nuclear factor κB transcriptional activation in neuroblastoma SH-SY5Y cells. Biochem J 406:215–221

Lin X, Wang YJ, Li Q, Hou YY, Hong MH, Cao YL, Chi ZQ, Liu JG (2009) Chronic high-dose morphine treatment promotes SH-SY5Y cell apoptosis via c-Jun N-terminal kinase-mediated activation of mitochondria-dependent pathway. FEBS J 276:2022–2036

Looney M, Doran P, Buggy DJ (2010) Effect of anesthetic technique on serum vascular endothelial growth factor C and transforming growth factor beta in women undergoing anesthesia and surgery for breast cancer. Anesthesiology 113:1118–1125

Lucchinetti E, Awad AE, Rahman M, Feng J, Lou PH, Zhang L, Ionescu L, Lemieux H, Thebaud B, Zaugg M (2012) Antiproliferative effects of local anesthetics on mesenchymal stem cells: potential implications for tumor spreading and wound healing. Anesthesiology 116:841–856

Luk K, Boatman S, Johnson KN, Dudek OA, Ristau N, Vang D, Nguyen J, Gupta K (2012) Influence of morphine on pericyte-endothelial interaction: implications for antiangiogenic therapy. J Oncol 2012:458385

Macfarlane GJ, McBeth J, Silman AJ (2001) Widespread body pain and mortality: prospective population based study. BMJ 323:662–665

Maneckjee R, Minna JD (1990) Opioid and nicotine receptors affect growth regulation of human lung cancer cell lines. Proc Natl Acad Sci USA 87:3294–3298

Maneckjee R, Minna JD (1994) Opioids induce while nicotine suppresses apoptosis in human lung cancer cells. Cell Growth Differ 5:1033–1040

Maneckjee R, Biswas R, Vonderhaar BK (1990) Binding of opioids to human MCF-7 breast cancer cells and their effects on growth. Cancer Res 50:2234–2238

Martucci C, Panerai AE, Sacerdote P (2004) Chronic fentanyl or buprenorphine infusion in the mouse: similar analgesic profile but different effects on immune responses. Pain 110:385–392

Mathew B, Lennon FE, Siegler J, Mirzapoiazova T, Mambetsariev N, Sammani S, Gerhold LM, LaRiviere PJ, Chen CT, Garcia JGN, Salgia R, Moss J, Singleton PA (2011) The novel role of the mu opioid receptor in lung cancer progression: a laboratory investigation. Anesth Analg 112:558–567

Mojadadi S, Jamali A, Khansarinejad B, Soleimanjahi H, Bamdad T (2009) Acute morphine administration reduces cell-mediated immunity and induces reactivation of latent herpes simplex virus type 1 in BALB/c mice. Cell Mol Immunol 6:111–116

Myles PS, Peyton P, Silbert B, Hunt J, Rigg JR, Sessler DI (2011) Perioperative epidural analgesia for major abdominal surgery for cancer and recurrence-free survival: randomised trial. BMJ 342:d1491

Nylund G, Pettersson A, Bengtsson C, Khorram-Manesh A, Nordgren S, Delbro DS (2008) Functional expression of mu-opioid receptors in the human colon cancer cell line, HT-29, and their localization in human colon. Dig Dis Sci 53:461–466

Ohara T, Itoh T, Takahashi M (2005) Immunosuppression by morphine-induced lymphocyte apoptosis: is it a real issue? Anesth Analg 101:1117–1122

Qin Y, Chen J, Li L, Liao CJ, Liang YB, Guan EJ, Xie YB (2012) Exogenous morphine inhibits human gastric cancer MGC-803 cell growth by cell cycle arrest and apoptosis induction. Asian Pac J Cancer Prev 13:1377–1382

Sasamura T, Nakamura S, Iida Y, Fujii H, Murata J, Saiki I, Nojima H, Kuraishi Y (2002) Morphine analgesia suppresses tumor growth and metastasis in a mouse model of cancer pain produced by orthotopic tumor inoculation. Eur J Pharmacol 441:185–191

Shavit Y, Ben-Eliyahu S, Zeidel A, Beilin B (2004) Effects of fentanyl on natural killer cell activity and on resistance to tumor metastasis in rats: dose and timing study. Neuroimmunomodulation 11:255–260

Singleton PA, Lingen MW, Fekete MJ, Garcia JGN, Moss J (2006) Methylnaltrexone inhibits opiate and VEGF-induced angiogenesis: role of receptor transactivation. Microvasc Res 72:3–11

Smith TJ, Staats PS, Deer T, Stearns LJ, Rauck RL, Boortz-Marx RL, Buchser E, Catala E, Bryce DA, Coyne PJ, Pool GE (2002) Randomized clinical trial of an implantable drug delivery system compared with comprehensive medical management for refractory cancer pain: impact on pain, drug-related toxicity, and survival. J Clin Oncol 20:4040–4049

Sueoka N, Sueoka E, Okabe S, Fujiki H (1996) Anti-cancer effects of morphine through inhibition of tumour necrosis factor-alpha release and mRNA expression. Carcinogenesis 17:2337–2341

Sueoka E, Sueoka N, Kai Y, Okabe S, Suganuma M, Kanematsu K, Yamamoto T, Fujiki H (1998) Anticancer activity of morphine and its synthetic derivative, KT-90, mediated through apoptosis and inhibition of NF-kappaB activation. Biochem Biophys Res Commun 252:566–570

Tegeder I, Grosch S, Schmidtko A, Haussler A, Schmidt H, Niederberger E, Scholich K, Geisslinger G (2003) G protein-independent G1 cell cycle block and apoptosis with morphine in adenocarcinoma cells: involvement of p53 phosphorylation. Cancer Res 63:1846–1852

Tsui BC, Rashiq S, Schopflocher D, Murtha A, Broemling S, Pillay J, Finucane BT (2010) Epidural anesthesia and cancer recurrence rates after radical prostatectomy. Can J Anaesth 57:107–112

Ustun F, Durmus-Altun G, Altaner S, Tuncbilek N, Uzal C, Berkarda S (2011) Evaluation of morphine effect on tumour angiogenesis in mouse breast tumour model, EATC. Med Oncol 28:1264–1272

Varadhan KK, Neal KR, Dejong CHC, Fearon KCH, Ljungqvist O, Lobo DN (2010) The enhanced recovery after surgery (ERAS) pathway for patients undergoing major elective open colorectal surgery: a meta-analysis of randomized controlled trials. Clin Nutr 29:434–440

Wuethrich PY, Hsu Schmitz SF, Kessler TM, Thalmann GN, Studer UE, Stueber F, Burkhard FC (2010) Potential influence of the anesthetic technique used during open radical prostatectomy on prostate cancer-related outcome: a retrospective study. Anesthesiology 113:570–576

Yin D, Woodruff M, Zhang Y, Whaley S, Miao J, Ferslew K, Zhao J, Stuart C (2006) Morphine promotes Jurkat cell apoptosis through pro-apoptotic FADD/P53 and anti-apoptotic PI3K/Akt/NF-kappaB pathways. J Neuroimmunol 174:101–107

Zagon IS, McLaughlin PJ (2003) Opioids and the apoptotic pathway in human cancer cells. Neuropeptides 37:79–88

Zagon IS, Rahn KA, McLaughlin PJ (2007) Opioids and migration, chemotaxis, invasion, and adhesion of human cancer cells. Neuropeptides 41:441–452

# Chapter 7
# Genetic Polymorphisms in the μ-Opioid Receptor Gene and Breast Cancer Survival

**Andrey V. Bortsov, Robert C. Millikan, Inna Belfer, Richard L. Boortz-Marx, Harendra Arora, and Samuel A. McLean**

**Abstract** Preclinical studies suggest that endogenous opioids and/or opioid medications may contribute to tumor growth. However, endogenous and exogenous opioids have not been modulated over time in cancer patients, who often need opioids for pain control. Most of the analgesic effect of opioids occurs through the activation of the μ-opioid receptor. The most common naturally occurring genetic variation of this receptor in humans is the so-called A118G mutation. Individuals with this mutation have been shown to have a reduced analgesic response to opioid medications. In a recent study, we used this naturally occurring genetic variation to look for evidence that endogenous and/or exogenous opioids influence tumor growth in humans. We hypothesized that if opioids do influence tumor growth, then cancer patients with the A118G mutation, *as a group*, should have longer survivals than those without it. Using data from the Carolina Breast Cancer Study, we found that, among 2,039 women diagnosed with breast cancer, the presence of A118G was associated with longer breast cancer specific survival. The protective effect of A118G was limited to invasive cases only and appeared to increase with the stage of cancer at diagnosis.

A.V. Bortsov, M.D., Ph.D. (✉) • R.L. Boortz-Marx, M.D. • H. Arora, M.B.B.S. •
S.A. McLean, M.D., M.P.H.
Department of Anesthesiology, University of North Carolina at Chapel Hill,
N2201 UNC Hospitals CB 7010, Chapel Hill, NC 27599-7010, USA
e-mail: abortsov@aims.unc.edu; rboortz-marx@aims.unc.edu; harora@aims.unc.edu;
smclean@aims.unc.edu

R.C. Millikan, DVM, Ph.D.
Department of Epidemiology, University of North Carolina at Chapel Hill,
Chapel Hill, NC 27599, USA
e-mail: millikan@email.unc.edu

I. Belfer, M.D., Ph.D.
Department of Anesthesiology, University of Pittsburg,
Pittsburgh, PA 15260, USA
e-mail: belferi@upmc.edu

M.-O. Parat (ed.), *Morphine and Metastasis*, DOI 10.1007/978-94-007-5678-6_7, 

This study did not assess whether opioid pain medications have any influence on cancer mortality. Moreover, the study was performed in African Americans and European Americans only, and requires replication.

**Keywords** μ-Opioid receptor • Allele • Breast cancer • Cancer survival • Endorphins • Exon • Intron • Linkage disequilibrium • Single nucleotide polymorphism

## Abbreviations

| | |
|---|---|
| DAMGO | [D-Ala2, N-MePhe4, Gly-ol]-enkephalin |
| *OPRM1* | μ-opioid receptor gene 1 |
| cAMP | adenosine 3′ 5′-cyclic monophosphate |
| ER | estrogen receptor |
| kb | kilobases |
| mRNA | messenger ribonucleic acid |
| NDI | National Death Index |
| SNP | single nucleotide polymorphism |
| SSN | social security number |

## 7.1 Introduction

μ-Opioid receptor activation by endogenous opioids (e.g. endorphins) or exogenous opioids (e.g. morphine) results in analgesia (Waldhoer et al. 2004). Importantly, in addition to this well known analgesic effect, μ-opioid receptor activation has other less well known effects that may influence tumor growth and cancer progression (Afsharimani et al. 2011). Stimulation of μ-opioid receptors on endothelial cells results in angiogenesis (Farooqui et al. 2007; Gupta et al. 2002; Poonawala et al. 2005; Singleton et al. 2006). In addition, opioids appear to suppress a number of aspects of immune system function, and some of these effects have been shown to be mediated by μ-opioid receptor activation (reviewed in Roy et al. 2011). For example, stimulation of μ-opioid receptors on immune cells reduces macrophage and lymphocyte proliferation and cytokine secretion (Roy et al. 1998, 2006; Szabo et al. 1993; Wang et al. 2008). Activation of μ-opioid receptors in brainstem regions modulates hypothalamic-adrenal-pituitary axis function and increases peripheral glucocorticoids (Bart et al. 2006), which may compromise immune function and promote tumor growth (Ben-Eliyahu 2003; Dietrich et al. 2009). Preclinical studies (Mathew et al. 2011; Boehncke et al. 2011) and limited human data (Cata et al. 2011) have implicated opioid pathways in the progression of several different types of cancers.

If μ-opioid receptor activation mediates processes which influence tumor growth, then naturally occurring genetic variations which affect μ-opioid receptor function would be expected to be associated with differences in cancer progression, and ultimately survival, in cancer patients.

### 7.1.1 μ-Opioid Receptor Gene

The μ-opioid receptor gene (*OPRM1*) is located on chromosome 6 and spans over 200 kb (Fig. 7.1). The most common transcript from this gene consists of exons 1–4 and is approximately 15 kb in length (Ide et al. 2005). New evidence suggests that *OPRM1* may have up to 18 exons that combine to multiple splice variants (Xu et al. 2009; Shabalina et al. 2009). Over 5,000 single nucleotide polymorphisms (SNPs) were identified in the *OPRM1* gene according to dbSNP database (http://www.ncbi.nlm.nih.gov/snp; accessed 03/04/2012).

A118G is the most common SNP in the coding region of the human μ-opioid receptor gene *OPRM1*, in which A at position 118 in exon 1 is replaced by G. This SNP results in the substitution of asparagine at position 40 with aspartate in the N-terminal domain, which removes one of five potential N-linked glycosylation sites of the receptor (Bond et al. 1998). The A118G allele frequency varies across populations, from 0.35 to 0.48 in Asians, 0.1 to 0.17 in Hispanics and European Americans, to as low as 0.04 in African Americans (Kreek et al. 2005). It has been shown using HapMap data that A118G may have undergone recent positive selection, i.e. an increase in allele frequency in the population when this allele confers a survival or reproductive advantage to the species (Pang et al. 2009). A118G may also inactivate three transcription factor binding sites (myogenin, RF1 and RFX1) and create a novel exon splicing enhancer site and creation of the new p53 binding site thus resulting in altered expression of μ-opioid receptor (Pang et al. 2009).

It has been shown that A118G in populations of European descent is located on the border of two haploblocks (Levran et al. 2011). The A118G allele is also part of a different haplogroup that includes several variants in the distal 5′-untranslated region that may have regulatory potential (Levran et al. 2011). In addition, in a recent study A118G was shown to be part of a six-SNP haplotype associated with pain sensitivity in healthy European American volunteers (Shabalina et al. 2009).

### 7.1.2 Potential Mechanisms of A118G Action

A118G has been shown to affect expression of the μ-opioid receptor. In a murine μ-opioid receptor gene, polymorphism A112G (which is equivalent to A118G in humans) was associated with reduced opioid receptor expression in some, but not all, brain regions. Additionally, the A112G SNP reduced receptor levels in more brain regions in male than in female mice (Wang et al. 2012). In humans, a postmortem study of individuals heterozygous on A118G found significant reductions in mRNA transcribed from the G118 allele (Zhang et al. 2005). A118G has also been shown to result in lower cell surface receptor binding site availability in cell lines expressing the μ-opioid receptor (Kroslak et al. 2007). Additionally, cell lines stably expressing μ-opioid receptor showed a decrease in agonist-mediated adenosine 3′ 5′-cyclic monophosphate (cAMP) signaling for morphine, methadone, and [D-Ala2, N-MePhe4, Gly-ol]-enkephalin (DAMGO), but not β-endorphin; this

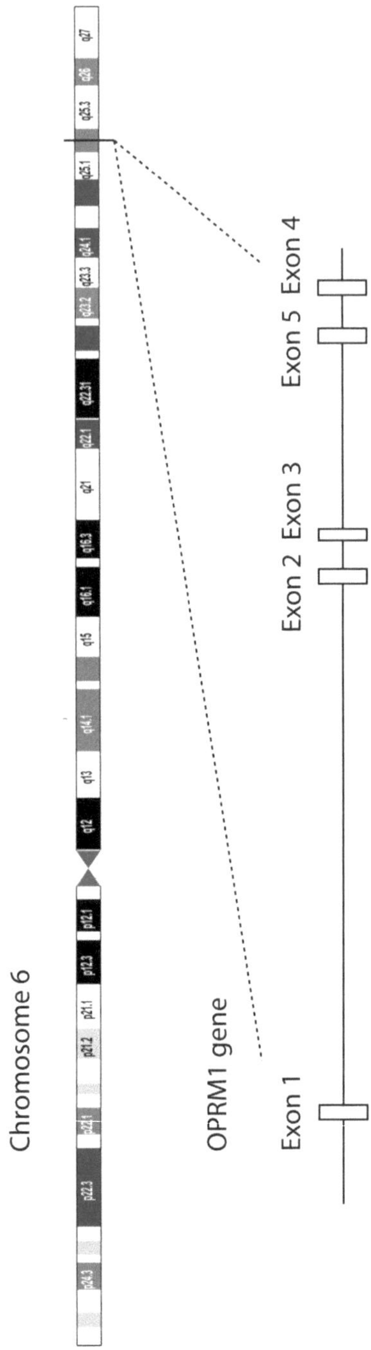


**Fig. 7.1** μ-Opioid receptor *OPRM1* gene. Adapted from ENSEMBL Genome Browser (www.ensembl.org)

effect was not seen in cell lines transiently expressing the receptor (Kroslak et al. 2007). The decrease in binding site availability was confirmed in another study; however, no alterations in binding affinity or signal transduction were detected in the G118 variant (Beyer et al. 2004).

Another proposed explanation of the A118G effect is that A118G reduces μ-opioid receptor N-glycosylation and protein stability (Huang et al. 2012). N-glycosylation of μ-opioid receptor is essential for proper presentation of the receptor on the plasma membrane (Kroslak et al. 2007).

Despite extensive research, the exact mechanism of A118G effect on the observed physiologic functions remains unknown.

### *7.1.3 A118G and Analgesia*

The G118 allele has been associated with reduced response to morphine or other opioids for patients receiving treatment for post-operative or chronic pain. In one study, the effect of morphine in cancer pain was significantly higher in AA homozygotes than in those carrying a G allele (Campa et al. 2008). In addition, among patients undergoing hysterectomy, patients homozygous for G118 required more morphine patient-controlled analgesia doses in the first 24 h after surgery to achieve adequate pain relief compared with patients homozygous for A118 (Chou et al. 2006). In another study of patients undergoing major open abdominal surgery under combined general and epidural anesthesia followed by continuous postoperative epidural analgesia with opioids, patients homozygous for the G allele required more analgesics during the first 24 h than AA homozygous and heterozygous patients (Hayashida et al. 2008). In G118 allele-carrying subjects, there was also a reduced potency of morphine-6-glucuronide (an active metabolite of morphine that has a greater analgesic potency but a reduced potency for respiratory depression) in eliciting an analgesic response, though there was no difference in morphine-6-glucuronide-induced respiratory depression (Romberg et al. 2005). In sum, evidence suggests that G allele carriers may require higher opioid doses to achieve adequate analgesia.

## 7.2 Genetic Evidence for the Involvement of the Opioid System in Cancer Progression in Humans

In a recent study (Bortsov et al. 2012), we explored the association between common polymorphisms in the μ-opioid receptor gene, including A118G, and breast cancer survival. With regard to A118G, we hypothesized that individuals with one or more copies of the (low-response) G allele would experience increased breast cancer survival.

### 7.2.1 Methods

The cohort of cancer female patients evaluated in our study came from the Carolina Breast Cancer Study; the methodology of the Carolina Breast Cancer Study is described in detail elsewhere (O'Brien et al. 2010). In brief, new cases of breast cancer from 24 counties of North Carolina diagnosed between 1993 and 2001 were identified using rapid case ascertainment. Written informed consent was obtained upon recruitment. An in-home interview was performed that included blood sample collection, information on menopausal status, and an assessment of other potential covariates. Ethnicity was determined by self-report questions during the interview; only African Americans or European Americans were eligible for recruitment. Data on estrogen receptor status and tumor stage at diagnosis were obtained from patient medical records. Subsequent patient survival outcomes were determined using National Death Index (NDI) data.

An NDI search was performed using the standard criteria as suggested in the *NDI User's Guide* (2010). An NDI record would match a submitted record if any of the following seven criteria are met: (1) social security number (SSN); (2) first and last name, exact month of birth, year of birth within 1 year; (3) last name, first initial and middle initial, exact month of birth, year of birth within 1 year; (4) first and last name, exact month of birth, exact day of birth; (5) last name, first initial and middle initial, exact month of birth, exact day of birth; (6) first name, father's surname, exact month of birth, exact year of birth; (7) for females only, first name, exact month and year of birth, and last name from the submitted record matching birth surname on the NDI record. As a result of the search, none, one, or more NDI records may be matched to a given submitted record. Besides the variables used in the seven matching criteria, the NDI search returned an indication of agreement for a number of other variables. After the search, each possible match record was assigned a probabilistic match score (the sum of the weights assigned to each of the variables used in the NDI record match) (Rogot et al. 1986). After scoring the potential matches, each record was categorized into one of five classes: Class 1 (exact match on SSN, first name, middle initial, last names, sex, state of birth, birth month and birth year); Class 2 (SSN matches on at least seven digits and one or more of the other items from Class 1 may not match); Class 3 (SSN unknown but eight or more of first name, middle initial, last name, birth day, birth month, birth year, sex, race, marital status, or state of birth match); Class 4 (Same as Class 3 but less than eight items match); Class 5 (SSN is known but doesn't match). All of Class 1 matches were considered to be true matches; all of the Class 5 matches were considered false matches. Records categorized into one of Classes 2, 3, or 4 were considered either true matches or false matches based on score cut-off points (44.5 for Class 2; 37.5 for Class 3; 32.5 for Class 4). The sensitivity of NDI search is estimated to be 98% and specificity approximately 100% (Rich-Edwards et al. 1994). Date of death and cause of death were obtained for each deceased individual. Cause of death was classified as breast cancer-specific if the first listed underlying cause of death had International Classification of Disease codes 174.9 (version 9) or 50.9 (version 10).

DNA was extracted from peripheral blood lymphocytes by standard methods using an automated Nucleic Acid Purification System ABI-DNA extractor (Applied Biosystems Inc., Foster City, CA), and subsequently stored prior to study analyses. For our study, we chose to examine the association between breast cancer survival and A118G SNP (rs1799971, located within the first exon) and five other informative SNPs within other parts of the μ-opioid receptor gene *OPRM1* (first intron (rs495491, rs563649), second intron (rs2075572), third intron (rs533586), and fifth exon (3′-untranslated region) (rs609148)) (Shabalina et al. 2009). Genotyping was performed using the TaqMan platform (Applied Biosystems Inc., Foster City, CA). Genotyping was repeated on a 10% random sample of participants. There was 100% call agreement between original and repeat genotyping. Institutional Review Board at the University of North Carolina at Chapel Hill (Chapel Hill, North Carolina, USA) approval was obtained prior to the data collection and genetic analyses.

The Carolina Breast Cancer Study was designed as a case–control study. In addition to women with breast cancer, population-based controls were selected using a Division of Motor Vehicles registry for women younger than 65 years and a Health Care Financing Administration (now the Centers for Medicare and Medicaid Services) registry for women 65–74 years of age. The sampling fractions were designed to insure frequency matching to cases by race and 5-year age group. In our study, healthy controls were also genotyped in order to assess Hardy-Weinberg equilibrium and linkage disequilibrium for the six genotypes evaluated. Controls were used for these analyses rather than cases to avoid potential selection bias (Salanti et al. 2005).

#### 7.2.1.1 Statistical Analyses

Descriptive statistics were obtained for socio-demographic and clinical characteristics of the sample. Individual SNP and genotype frequencies for each locus were evaluated. Hardy–Weinberg equilibrium and linkage disequilibrium between loci were evaluated in healthy participants from the Carolina Breast Cancer Study control group using Haploview software (Barrett et al. 2005).

For the purpose of survival analyses, individuals with breast cancer living at December 31, 2006 and individuals who died of causes other than breast cancer were censored. Breast cancer-specific survival was estimated using Kaplan-Meier method, stratified by ethnicity and stage at diagnosis. The log-rank test was used to compare survival curves between genotype groups. Bonferroni correction was applied to the significance level for the six genotypes assessed to preserve an overall false positive rate of $\alpha = 0.05$. Within genotype A118G, subgroup analyses stratified by ethnicity and cancer stage were performed using significance level $\alpha = 0.05$.

Cox proportional hazards regression models were used to evaluate the effect of genotype on breast cancer-specific survival, adjusted for potential confounders. The proportional hazards assumption was tested using log-log survival plots and the Schoenfeld residuals approach (Kleinbaum and Klein 2005). All analyses, unless otherwise noted, were performed using SAS (version 9.2, SAS Institute Inc., Cary, NC).

**Table 7.1** Characteristics of the Carolina Breast Cancer Study cases (Bortsov et al. 2012)

| | n=2,039 |
|---|---|
| Age, years | |
| Mean (SD) | 51.9 (11.7) |
| Range | 23–74 |
| Ethnicity, n (%) | |
| African American | 766 (38) |
| European American | 1,273 (62) |
| Menopausal status, n (%) | |
| Premenopausal | 912 (45) |
| Postmenopausal | 1,127 (55) |
| Stage at diagnosis, n (%)[a] | |
| *In situ* | 451 (23) |
| Invasive: | |
| I | 635 (33) |
| II | 663 (34) |
| III | 153 (8) |
| IV | 44 (2) |
| Estrogen receptor status, n (%) | |
| Positive | 1,045 (59) |
| Negative | 719 (41) |
| Follow up period, years | |
| Median | 9.0 |
| Range | 0.4–13.7 |

[a] American Joint Committee on Cancer criteria
*SD* standard deviation

### 7.2.2 Results

Characteristics of the breast cancer patient cohort are shown in Table 7.1. A total of 2,039 women (766 African Americans and 1,273 European Americans) were included in the analyses. Invasive breast cancer cases constituted 77%. Median follow up period was 9 years. All six polymorphisms were genotyped with success rates $\geq 98\%$. All six polymorphisms were in Hardy–Weinberg equilibrium and moderate-to-high linkage disequilibrium (Fig. 7.2).

After Bonferroni correction for multiple comparisons, the A118G genotype was significantly associated with breast cancer-specific mortality (Table 7.2). Breast cancer-specific mortality was reduced in women with one or two copies of the G-allele (Table 7.2). Analyses stratified by ethnicity, although not reaching statistical significance, revealed the effect for A118G of the same direction in both African Americans and European Americans (Table 7.3). Women with at least one copy of G allele had lower mortality than those with A/A genotype (Table 7.3). Analysis stratified by stage at diagnosis (Table 7.4, Fig. 7.3) revealed that the observed effect of A118G was limited to invasive cases only (stages I–IV), with effect size increasing

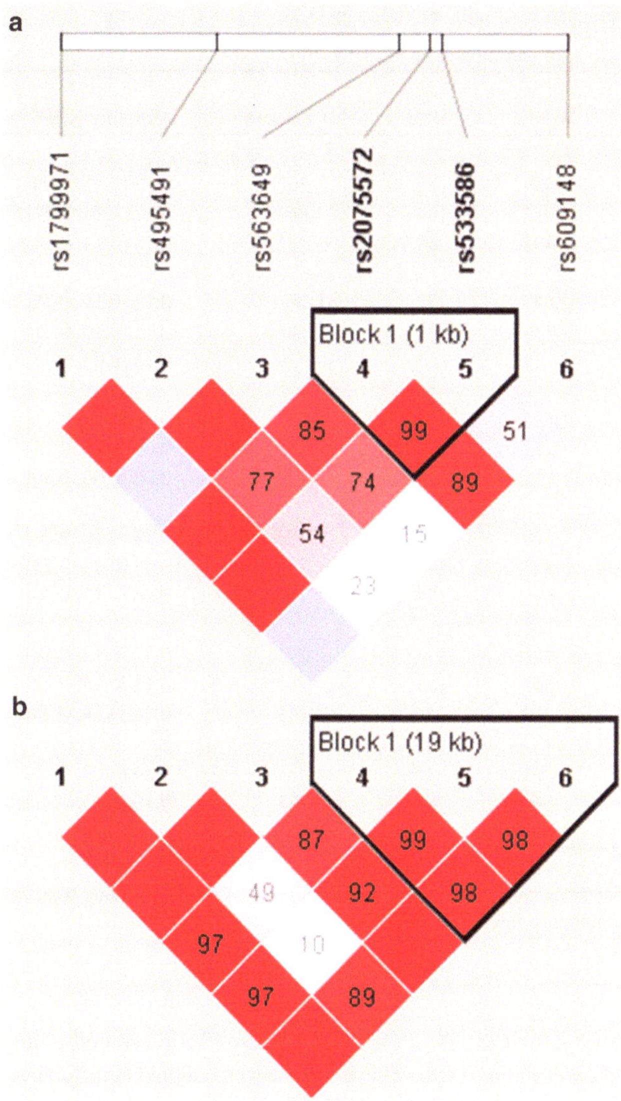


**Fig. 7.2** Linkage disequilibrium plots for 679 African American controls (**a**) and 1,131 European American controls (**b**). Color represents D′ values (dark red = high inter-SNP D′; blue = statistically ambiguous D′; white = low inter-SNP D′), and $r^2$ values are contained within blocks. Block definitions are calculated using the Gabriel et al. method (Gabriel et al. 2002). Reproduced with permission from (Bortsov et al. 2012)

with cancer stage at diagnosis. No other polymorphisms were associated with breast cancer survival (Table 7.2).

A118G genotype was also associated with breast cancer stage at diagnosis. Women who presented at a more advanced stage (III–IV) were less likely to have

**Table 7.2** Breast cancer-specific mortality by OPRM1 genotype (Bortsov et al. 2012)

| | All participants (n=2,039) | | | | |
|---|---|---|---|---|---|
| *OPRM1* genotype | n | Died | Censored | Mortality [CI][a,b] | p-value[c] |
| rs2075572 | | | | | |
| C/C | 589 | 85 | 502 | 0.15 [0.12, 0.20] | 0.57 |
| C/G | 1,012 | 164 | 844 | 0.17 [0.14, 0.21] | |
| G/G | 404 | 69 | 335 | 0.18 [0.14, 0.24] | |
| rs563649 | | | | | |
| C/C | 1,647 | 272 | 1,371 | 0.18 [0.15, 0.20] | 0.46 |
| C/T | 339 | 46 | 290 | 0.15 [0.10, 0.21] | |
| T/T | 23 | 3 | 20 | 0.13 [0.03, 0.47] | |
| rs1799971 | | | | | |
| A/A | 1,682 | 291 | 1,386 | 0.18 [0.16, 0.21] | <0.001 |
| A/G | 323 | 26 | 295 | 0.09 [0.05, 0.15] | |
| G/G | 22 | 1 | 21 | 0.05 [0.00, 0.50] | |
| rs533586 | | | | | |
| C/C | 220 | 37 | 183 | 0.18 [0.12, 0.26] | 0.88 |
| C/T | 907 | 147 | 758 | 0.18 [0.14, 0.21] | |
| T/T | 891 | 134 | 752 | 0.16 [0.13, 0.20] | |
| rs495491 | | | | | |
| A/A | 901 | 128 | 771 | 0.15 [0.12, 0.19] | 0.13 |
| A/G | 847 | 141 | 702 | 0.18 [0.15, 0.22] | |
| G/G | 269 | 50 | 218 | 0.20 [0.14, 0.28] | |
| rs609148 | | | | | |
| A/A | 94 | 13 | 81 | 0.14 [0.07, 0.27] | 0.44 |
| A/G | 640 | 95 | 543 | 0.16 [0.13, 0.21] | |
| G/G | 1,265 | 209 | 1,051 | 0.18 [0.15, 0.21] | |

[a] Ten-year mortality estimated using Kaplan–Meier method
[b] Confidence intervals are Bonferroni-adjusted (alpha=0.0083); Log–Log transform was used to compute the confidence intervals for the survivor function
[c] Log-rank test

one or more copies of the G allele than women who presented at an earlier stage (I–II) or with carcinoma *in situ*. These differences reached significance in European Americans (Cochran–Armitage trend test p=0.046), but not in African Americans (p=0.53) (Fig. 7.4). A118G was not associated with estrogen receptor status (data not shown).

Because the results from the crude and stratified survival analyses suggest that the effect of A118G genotype is a linear function of the number of G alleles, we ran a set of Cox proportional hazard regression models with the predictor variable representing the number of G alleles at A118G, a so called additive genetic model. The proportional hazard assumption was violated for cancer stage at diagnosis (p=0.005). The full Cox model included the interaction terms between A118G genotype and stage and A118G genotype and ethnicity. None of these interaction terms appeared significant (data not shown) and therefore were excluded from further models.

**Table 7.3** Breast cancer-specific mortality by OPRM1 genotype A118G, stratified by ethnicity (Bortsov et al. 2012)

| | A118G genotype | n | Died | Censored | Mortality [95%CI][a] | p-value[b] |
|---|---|---|---|---|---|---|
| African Americans (n=766) | A/A | 728 | 176 | 552 | 0.26 [0.23, 0.29] | 0.31 |
| | A/G | 34 | 5 | 29 | 0.15 [0.07, 0.33] | |
| | G/G | 2 | 0 | 2 | 0.00 [NE] | |
| European Americans (n=1,273) | A/A | 954 | 120 | 834 | 0.13 [0.11, 0.15] | 0.070 |
| | A/G | 289 | 23 | 266 | 0.08 [0.05, 0.13] | |
| | G/G | 20 | 1 | 19 | 0.05 [0.01, 0.32] | |

[a] Ten-year mortality estimated using Kaplan–Meier method; Log-Log transform was used to compute the confidence limits for the survivor function
[b] Log-rank test
*NE* non-estimable, *CI* confidence interval

**Table 7.4** Breast cancer-specific mortality by *OPRM1* A118G genotype, stratified by stage at diagnosis (Bortsov et al. 2012)

| Stage at diagnosis | A118G genotype | n | Died | Censored | Mortality [95%CI][a] | p-value[b] |
|---|---|---|---|---|---|---|
| Carcinoma *in situ* | A/A | 350 | 6 | 344 | 0.03 [0.01, 0.08] | 0.037 |
| | A/G | 90 | 0 | 90 | 0.00 [NE] | |
| | G/G | 9 | 1 | 8 | 0.11 [0.02, 0.57] | |
| Stage I | A/A | 522 | 42 | 479 | 0.09 [0.06, 0.11] | 0.71 |
| | A/G | 110 | 5 | 103 | 0.05 [0.02, 0.11] | |
| | G/G | 2 | 0 | 2 | 0.00 [NE] | |
| Stage II | A/A | 554 | 127 | 423 | 0.24 [0.21, 0.28] | 0.075 |
| | A/G | 91 | 15 | 76 | 0.18 [0.11, 0.28] | |
| | G/G | 10 | 0 | 10 | 0.00 [NE] | |
| Stage III–IV | A/A | 182 | 100 | 82 | 0.58 [0.51, 0.66] | 0.085 |
| | A/G | 14 | 4 | 10 | 0.29 [0.12, 0.59] | |
| | G/G | – | – | – | – | |

[a] Ten-year mortality estimated using Kaplan-Meier method; the Log-Log transform was used to compute the confidence limits for the survivor function
[b] Log-rank test
*NE* non-estimable

Because inclusion of postmenopausal and estrogen receptor (ER) status did not change the hazard ratio estimates for A118G genotype, and because A118 genotype was associated with cancer stage at presentation, the final model included only age and ethnicity (Table 7.5, Model 1). The association between A118G genotype and breast cancer survival remained statistically significant (p=0.006).

As a sensitivity analysis we repeated the survival analyses using all-cause mortality as an outcome. The results yielded the same findings (data not shown).

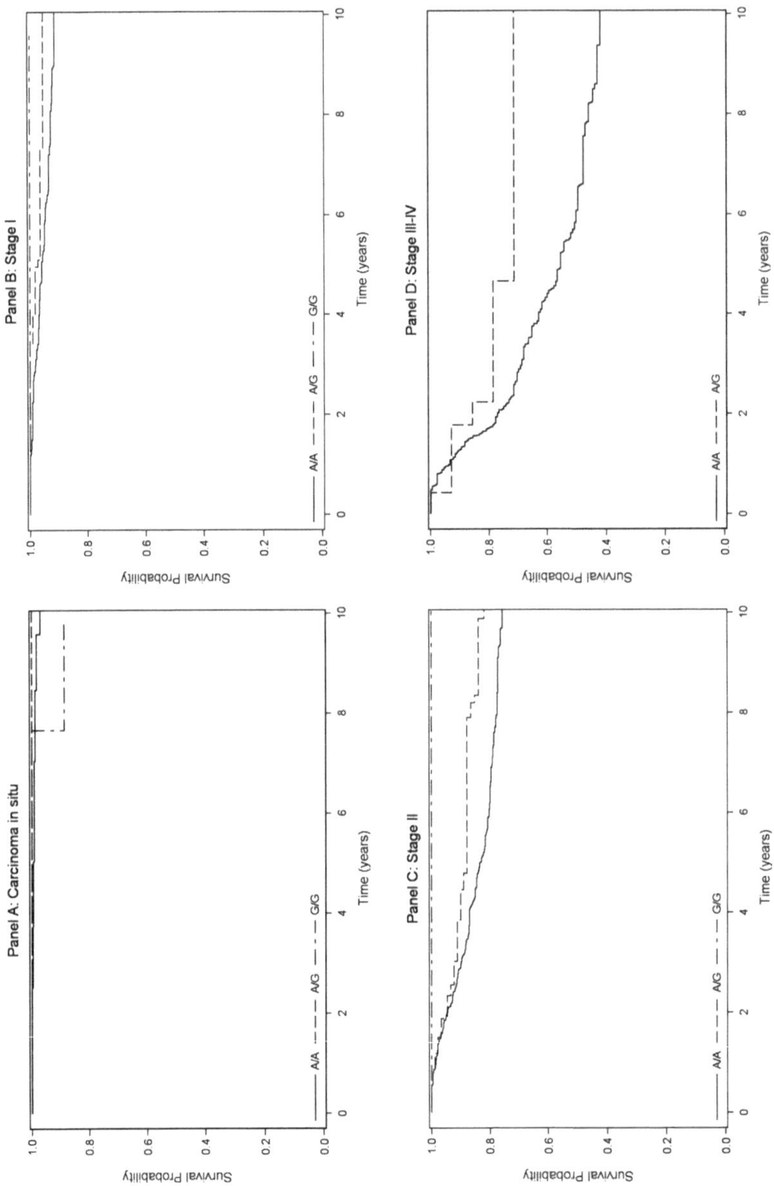


**Fig. 7.3** Kaplan-Meier plots by A118G (rs1799971) genotype and breast cancer stage at diagnosis (Bortsov et al. 2012)

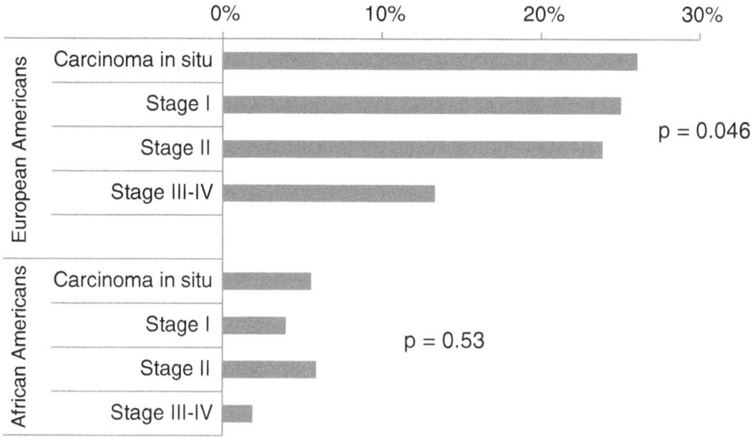


**Fig. 7.4** Proportion of A/G+G/G genotype by breast cancer stage in African Americans and European Americans (p-values are from Cochran–Armitage trend test)

**Table 7.5** Cox proportional hazards regression analysis for A118G genotype and invasive breast cancer survival (Bortsov et al. 2012)[a]

| | A118G genotype | HR | [95%CI] | p-value |
|---|---|---|---|---|
| Model 1[b] | A/A | | Reference | |
| | A/G | 0.57 | [0.38, 0.85] | 0.006 |
| | G/G | 0.32 | [0.22, 0.49] | |

[a] Additive genetic model was used, where the predictor variable was the number of A alleles at A118G (A/A = 0, A/G = 1, G/G = 2)
[b] Adjusted for age and race

## 7.2.3 *Discussion*

In our recent study breast cancer-specific mortality was significantly reduced in patients with a genetic variant in the μ-opioid receptor which reduces opioid response (Bortsov et al. 2012). Ten-year mortality was reduced in patients with at least one variant G allele at A118G. The protective effect of this polymorphism was limited to invasive cases only and appeared to increase with the stage at diagnosis. Decreased mortality with one or more G alleles was observed in both African Americans and European Americans, although the association did not reach statistical significance in stratified analyses. Having one or more G alleles was also associated with having less advanced disease at diagnosis.

Our results are consistent with a post-hoc analysis of data from a longitudinal study of traditional high dose systemic opioid treatment vs. opioid treatment delivered directly into the intrathecal space (low systemic opioid exposure) via an implantable drug delivery system (Smith et al. 2002). This trial was designed to assess symptomatic outcomes, but a post-hoc analysis, although statistically non-significant, suggested increased survival in the implantable drug delivery system group at 6 months (54% vs. 37%, p=0.06) (Smith et al. 2002).

Other studies have examined the effect of reduced opioid exposure during the perioperative period on cancer outcomes, with mixed effects. Two retrospective studies of cancer patients found a reduced risk of tumor recurrence and metastasis in cases where an opioid-sparing perioperative regimen was used (Biki et al. 2008; Exadaktylos et al. 2006). Another study observed this benefit only in patients 65 years of age or older (Gottschalk et al. 2010), and a secondary analysis of a randomized controlled study showed no difference (Tsui et al. 2010). If opioids influence tumor growth in an ongoing manner via direct (e.g. angiogenic) and/or indirect (immune function) mechanisms, then combined interventions which reduce both perioperative opioid exposure and longitudinal opioid exposure after hospital discharge (e.g., via peripherally acting opioid antagonists or implantable drug delivery systems) may achieve the most benefit.

In our study, the presence of a G allele at A118G appeared to result in improved survival in both European Americans and African Americans, although the association did not reach statistical significance in stratified analyses (Bortsov et al. 2012). Of note, available data suggests that the G allele is less prevalent in African Americans than in European Americans (minor allele frequency of 0.04 vs. 0.16, HapMap database). If having a G allele is indeed associated with increased breast cancer survival, then ethnic differences at A118G could contribute to the reduced breast cancer survival observed in African Americans (Holmes et al. 2010; Grann et al. 2006).

A limitation of our study was that data on treatment, including opioid intake among study participants, was not available. Therefore, we were unable to assess the extent to which any effect of opioids on cancer survival is mediated by endogenous vs. exogenous opioids. However, limited available evidence suggests that endogenous opioids may play an important role. A preclinical study found that baseline levels of endogenous opioids were elevated more than twofold in animals with cancer compared to controls (Lee et al. 2009), suggesting that cancer patients may experience chronic increases in endogenous opioids due to pain, stress, or other causes. In addition, a recent study found that, unlike wild-type mice, μ-opioid receptor-knockout mice exhibited no tumor growth after injection of Lewis lung carcinoma cells (Mathew et al. 2011). No exogenous opioids were received by mice in either group, suggesting that an angiogenic or tumor growth promoting effect was facilitated by stimulation of the μ-opioid receptor by endogenous opioids alone.

As with any gene association study, another limitation of our study is that it was impossible to know if differences in breast cancer survival were actually due to the A118G mutation. This mutation has been shown to result in reduced transcription (Zhang et al. 2005) and reduced cellular response to μ-opioid receptor binding (Ray et al. 2011). This demonstrated functional consequence increases the possibility that the A118G polymorphism may itself cause the biological changes which result in differences in breast cancer survival. However, it may be that the observed association is due to another genetic variation or variations that are associated with A118G (Shabalina et al. 2009).

In addition, another limitation of our study is that it included European American and African American patients only, and assessed only patients with breast cancer. Further studies are needed to confirm the association between A118G and cancer survival in Breast Cancer patients in European Americans and African Americans, and to assess the influence of A118G in other cancer types and in other ethnicities. Importantly, evidence from mechanistic studies in humans suggests that important differences in the influence of genetic variants such as the A118G polymorphism across other ethnicities may exist (e.g. Asians vs. European Americans (Hernandez-Avila et al. 2007)), perhaps in part due to differences in linkage disequilibrium between A118G and other functional polymorphisms in *OPRM1* or genetic differences influencing the function of physiologic systems which interact with opioid systems (Hernandez-Avila et al. 2007).

Our study used the first underlying cause of death listed in the NDI to determine breast cancer-specific mortality. Evidence suggests that variability may exist in the choice of the condition listed first as the cause of death in the NDI (Maynard et al. 2008). However, an analysis using all-cause mortality yielded the same findings.

Finally, G/G genotype at A118G was uncommon in the studied population, and only one death was observed among 22 participants with this genotype. Therefore, mortality estimates for this group are imprecise as evident from the wide confidence intervals (Table 7.2). Therefore, one should be cautious in making any conclusions regarding the presence of "dose–response" relationship between the number of G alleles at A118G and breast cancer mortality.

To our knowledge, the described study was the first to examine the association between genetic polymorphisms influencing the function of opioid pathways and cancer survival (Singleton and Moss 2010; Durieux 2009). Such studies are one useful means of examining the possible influence of opioid pathways on cancer survival in patients in whom withholding opioids would be unethical. The results of our study provide support for the hypothesis that endogenous and/or exogenous opioids, acting via the μ-opioid receptor, may influence cancer outcomes.

## References


Afsharimani B, Cabot P, Parat MO (2011) Morphine and tumor growth and metastasis. Cancer Metastasis Rev 30(2):225–238

Barrett JC, Fry B, Maller J, Daly MJ (2005) Haploview: analysis and visualization of LD and haplotype maps. Bioinformatics 21(2):263–265

Bart G, LaForge KS, Borg L, Lilly C, Ho A, Kreek MJ (2006) Altered levels of basal cortisol in healthy subjects with a 118G allele in exon 1 of the Mu opioid receptor gene. Neuropsychopharmacology 31(10):2313–2317

Ben-Eliyahu S (2003) The promotion of tumor metastasis by surgery and stress: immunological basis and implications for psychoneuroimmunology. Brain Behav Immun 17(Suppl 1):S27–36

Beyer A, Koch T, Schroder H, Schulz S, Hollt V (2004) Effect of the A118G polymorphism on binding affinity, potency and agonist-mediated endocytosis, desensitization, and resensitization of the human mu-opioid receptor. J Neurochem 89(3):553–560

Biki B, Mascha E, Moriarty DC, Fitzpatrick JM, Sessler DI, Buggy DJ (2008) Anesthetic technique for radical prostatectomy surgery affects cancer recurrence: a retrospective analysis. Anesthesiology 109(2):180–187

Boehncke S, Hardt K, Schadendorf D, Henschler R, Boehncke WH, Duthey B (2011) Endogenous mu-opioid peptides modulate immune response towards malignant melanoma. Exp Dermatol 20(1):24–28

Bond C, LaForge KS, Tian M, Melia D, Zhang S, Borg L, Gong J, Schluger J, Strong JA, Leal SM, Tischfield JA, Kreek MJ, Yu L (1998) Single-nucleotide polymorphism in the human mu opioid receptor gene alters beta-endorphin binding and activity: possible implications for opiate addiction. Proc Natl Acad Sci U S A 95(16):9608–9613

Bortsov AV, Millikan RC, Belfer I, Boortz-Marx RL, Arora H, McLean SA (2012) Mu-opioid receptor gene A118G polymorphism predicts survival in patients with breast cancer. Anesthesiology 116(4):896–902

Campa D, Gioia A, Tomei A, Poli P, Barale R (2008) Association of ABCB1/MDR1 and OPRM1 gene polymorphisms with morphine pain relief. Clin Pharmacol Ther 83(4):559–566

Cata JP, Gottumukkala V, Sessler DI (2011) How regional analgesia might reduce postoperative cancer recurrence. Eur J Pain Suppl 5(2):345–355

Chou WY, Wang CH, Liu PH, Liu CC, Tseng CC, Jawan B (2006) Human opioid receptor A118G polymorphism affects intravenous patient-controlled analgesia morphine consumption after total abdominal hysterectomy. Anesthesiology 105(2):334–337

Dietrich K, Schned A, Fortuny J, Heaney J, Marsit C, Kelsey KT, Karagas MR (2009) Glucocorticoid therapy and risk of bladder cancer. Br J Cancer 101(8):1316–1320

Durieux ME (2009) Does anesthetic management affect cancer outcome. APSF Newsl 23:49–51

Exadaktylos AK, Buggy DJ, Moriarty DC, Mascha E, Sessler DI (2006) Can anesthetic technique for primary breast cancer surgery affect recurrence or metastasis? Anesthesiology 105(4):660–664

Farooqui M, Li Y, Rogers T, Poonawala T, Griffin RJ, Song CW, Gupta K (2007) COX-2 inhibitor celecoxib prevents chronic morphine-induced promotion of angiogenesis, tumour growth, metastasis and mortality, without compromising analgesia. Br J Cancer 97(11):1523–1531

Gabriel SB, Schaffner SF, Nguyen H, Moore JM, Roy J, Blumenstiel B, Higgins J, DeFelice M, Lochner A, Faggart M (2002) The structure of haplotype blocks in the human genome. Science 296(5576):2225

Gottschalk A, Ford JG, Regelin CC, You J, Mascha EJ, Sessler DI, Durieux ME, Nemergut EC (2010) Association between epidural analgesia and cancer recurrence after colorectal cancer surgery. Anesthesiology 113(1):27–34

Grann V, Troxel AB, Zojwalla N, Hershman D, Glied SA, Jacobson JS (2006) Regional and racial disparities in breast cancer-specific mortality. Soc Sci Med 62(2):337–347

Gupta K, Kshirsagar S, Chang L, Schwartz R, Law PY, Yee D, Hebbel RP (2002) Morphine stimulates angiogenesis by activating proangiogenic and survival-promoting signaling and promotes breast tumor growth. Cancer Res 62(15):4491–4498

Hayashida M, Nagashima M, Satoh Y, Katoh R, Tagami M, Ide S, Kasai S, Nishizawa D, Ogai Y, Hasegawa J, Komatsu H, Sora I, Fukuda K, Koga H, Hanaoka K, Ikeda K (2008) Analgesic requirements after major abdominal surgery are associated with OPRM1 gene polymorphism genotype and haplotype. Pharmacogenomics 9(11):1605–1616

Hernandez-Avila CA, Covault J, Wand G, Zhang H, Gelernter J, Kranzler HR (2007) Population-specific effects of the Asn40Asp polymorphism at the mu-opioid receptor gene (OPRM1) on HPA-axis activation. Pharmacogenet Genomics 17(12):1031–1038

Holmes L Jr, Opara F, Hossain J (2010) A five-year breast cancer-specific survival disadvantage of African American women. Afr J Reprod Health 14(3):195–200

Huang P, Chen C, Mague SD, Blendy JA, Liu-Chen LY (2012) A common single nucleotide polymorphism A118G of the mu opioid receptor alters its N-glycosylation and protein stability. Biochem J 441(1):379–386

Ide S, Han W, Kasai S, Hata H, Sora I, Ikeda K (2005) Characterization of the 3′ untranslated region of the human mu-opioid receptor (MOR-1) mRNA. Gene 364:139–145

Kleinbaum DG, Klein M (2005) Survival analysis: a self-learning text. Springer, New York

Kreek MJ, Bart G, Lilly C, LaForge KS, Nielsen DA (2005) Pharmacogenetics and human molecular genetics of opiate and cocaine addictions and their treatments. Pharmacol Rev 57(1):1–26

Kroslak T, Laforge KS, Gianotti RJ, Ho A, Nielsen DA, Kreek MJ (2007) The single nucleotide polymorphism A118G alters functional properties of the human mu opioid receptor. J Neurochem 103(1):77–87

Lee HJ, Lee JH, Lee EO, Kim KH, Lee KS, Lee CH, Nam DW, Kim SH, Ahn KS (2009) Substance P and beta endorphin mediate electroacupuncture induced analgesic activity in mouse cancer pain model. Acupunct Electrother Res 34(1–2):27–40

Levran O, Awolesi O, Linzy S, Adelson M, Kreek MJ (2011) Haplotype block structure of the genomic region of the mu opioid receptor gene. J Hum Genet 56(2):147–155

Mathew B, Lennon FE, Siegler J, Mirzapoiazova T, Mambetsariev N, Sammani S, Gerhold LM, LaRiviere PJ, Chen CT, Garcia JG, Salgia R, Moss J, Singleton PA (2011) The novel role of the mu opioid receptor in lung cancer progression: a laboratory investigation. Anesth Analg 112(3):558–567

Maynard C, Lowy E, McDonell M, Fihn SD (2008) Cause of death in Washington state veterans hospitalized with acute coronary syndromes in the veterans health administration. Population Health Metrics 6(1):3

*NDI User's Guide* (2010) CDC/National Center for Health Statistics. http://www.cdc.gov/nchs/data_access/ndi/ndi_user_guide.htm. Accessed May 9 2010

O'Brien KM, Cole SR, Tse CK, Perou CM, Carey LA, Foulkes WD, Dressler LG, Geradts J, Millikan RC (2010) Intrinsic breast tumor subtypes, race, and long-term survival in the Carolina Breast Cancer Study. Clin Cancer Res 16(24):6100–6110

Pang GS, Wang J, Wang Z, Goh C, Lee CG (2009) The G allele of SNP E1/A118G at the mu-opioid receptor gene locus shows genomic evidence of recent positive selection. Pharmacogenomics 10(7):1101–1109

Poonawala T, Levay-Young BK, Hebbel RP, Gupta K (2005) Opioids heal ischemic wounds in the rat. Wound Repair Regen 13(2):165–174

Ray R, Ruparel K, Newberg A, Wileyto EP, Loughead JW, Divgi C, Blendy JA, Logan J, Zubieta JK, Lerman C (2011) Human Mu Opioid Receptor (OPRM1 A118G) polymorphism is associated with brain mu-opioid receptor binding potential in smokers. Proc Natl Acad Sci U S A 108(22):9268–9273

Rich-Edwards JW, Corsano KA, Stampfer MJ (1994) Test of the national death index and Equifax nationwide death search. Am J Epidemiol 140(11):1016–1019

Rogot E, Sorlie P, Johnson NJ (1986) Probabilistic methods in matching census samples to the National Death Index. J Chronic Dis 39(9):719–734

Romberg RR, Olofsen E, Bijl H, Taschner PE, Teppema LJ, Sarton EY, van Kleef JW, Dahan A (2005) Polymorphism of mu-opioid receptor gene (OPRM1:c.118A>G) does not protect against opioid-induced respiratory depression despite reduced analgesic response. Anesthesiology 102(3):522–530

Roy S, Barke RA, Loh HH (1998) MU-opioid receptor-knockout mice: role of [mu]-opioid receptor in morphine mediated immune functions. Molecular brain research 61(1–2):190–194

Roy S, Wang J, Kelschenbach J, Koodie L, Martin J (2006) Modulation of immune function by morphine: implications for susceptibility to infection. J Neuroimmune Pharmacol 1(1):77–89

Roy S, Ninkovic J, Banerjee S, Charboneau RG, Das S, Dutta R, Kirchner VA, Koodie L, Ma J, Meng J (2011) Opioid drug abuse and modulation of immune function: consequences in the susceptibility to opportunistic infections. J Neuroimmune Pharmacol 6(4):442–65

Salanti G, Amountza G, Ntzani EE, Ioannidis JP (2005) Hardy-Weinberg equilibrium in genetic association studies: an empirical evaluation of reporting, deviations, and power. Eur J Hum Genet 13(7):840–848

Shabalina SA, Zaykin DV, Gris P, Ogurtsov AY, Gauthier J, Shibata K, Tchivileva IE, Belfer I, Mishra B, Kiselycznyk C, Wallace MR, Staud R, Spiridonov NA, Max MB, Goldman D, Fillingim RB, Maixner W, Diatchenko L (2009) Expansion of the human mu-opioid receptor gene architecture: novel functional variants. Hum Mol Genet 18(6):1037–1051

Singleton PA, Moss J (2010) Effect of perioperative opioids on cancer recurrence: a hypothesis. Future Oncol 6(8):1237–1242
Singleton PA, Lingen MW, Fekete MJ, Garcia JG, Moss J (2006) Methylnaltrexone inhibits opiate and VEGF-induced angiogenesis: role of receptor transactivation. Microvasc Res 72(1–2):3–11
Smith TJ, Staats PS, Deer T, Stearns LJ, Rauck RL, Boortz-Marx RL, Buchser E, Catala E, Bryce DA, Coyne PJ, Pool GE (2002) Randomized clinical trial of an implantable drug delivery system compared with comprehensive medical management for refractory cancer pain: impact on pain, drug-related toxicity, and survival. J Clin Oncol 20(19):4040–4049
Szabo I, Rojavin M, Bussiere JL, Eisenstein TK, Adler MW, Rogers TJ (1993) Suppression of peritoneal macrophage phagocytosis of Candida albicans by opioids. J Pharmacol Exp Ther 267(2):703–706
Tsui BCH, Rashiq S, Schopflocher D, Murtha A, Broemling S, Pillay J, Finucane BT (2010) Epidural anesthesia and cancer recurrence rates after radical prostatectomy. Can J Anesth/J Can D'anesth 57(2):107–112
Waldhoer M, Bartlett SE, Whistler JL (2004) Opioid receptors. Annu Rev Biochem 73:953–990
Wang J, Barke RA, Ma J, Charboneau R, Roy S (2008) Opiate abuse, innate immunity, and bacterial infectious diseases. Arch Immunol Ther Exp 56(5):299–309
Wang YJ, Huang P, Ung A, Blendy JA, Liu-Chen LY (2012) Reduced expression of the mu opioid receptor in some, but not all, brain regions in mice with Oprm1 A112G. Neuroscience 205:178–184
Xu J, Xu M, Hurd YL, Pasternak GW, Pan YX (2009) Isolation and characterization of new exon 11-associated N-terminal splice variants of the human mu opioid receptor gene. J Neurochem 108(4):962–972
Zhang Y, Wang D, Johnson AD, Papp AC, Sadee W (2005) Allelic expression imbalance of human mu opioid receptor (OPRM1) caused by variant A118G. J Biol Chem 280(38):32618–32624

# Chapter 8
# Anaesthetic and Pain Management Technique in Long Term Cancer Outcome – Benefits of Regional Anaesthesia and Analgesia in the Context of Cancer Surgery

**Daniel M. Pöpping, Manuel Wenk, and Stephan A. Schug**

**Abstract** There has been an assumption, that the pharmacological effects of local anaesthetic agents and/or the analgesic benefits of regional anaesthesia and analgesia might lead to a reduction of cancer recurrence and/or metastases after cancer surgery. These benefits over general anaesthesia and opioid-based postoperative analgesia were claimed in particular with use of epidural techniques by retrospective studies. However, other retrospective and a number of prospective studies have not confirmed this impression in favour of epidural techniques. Similarly, there are inconclusive results with regard to the use of peripheral nerve blocks including paravertebral blocks and the use of spinal anaesthesia. Despite the theoretical potential of local anaesthetics and regional techniques, supported by in-vitro and animal studies, the current clinical situation is equivocal and further well-designed prospective studies are required to address this issue definitively.

**Keywords** Analgesia • Cancer surgery • Epidural • Opioid • Paravertebral block • Regional anaesthesia

D.M. Pöpping, M.D. • M. Wenk, M.D.
Department of Anaesthesiology and Intensive Care, Münster University Hospital, Albert-Schweitzer-Campus 1, Gebäude A1, 48149 Münster, Germany
e-mail: poppind@uni-muenster.de; manuelwenk@mac.com

S.A. Schug, M.D., FANZCA, FFPMANZCA (✉)
Department of Anaesthesiology, Pharmacology and Anaesthesiology Unit, School of Medicine and Pharmacology, University of Western Australia, Perth, WA 6847, Australia

Royal Perth Hospital, UWA Anaesthesia, Level 2, MRF Building G Block, GPO Box X2213, Perth, WA 6847, Australia
e-mail: stephan.schug@uwa.edu.au

M.-O. Parat (ed.), *Morphine and Metastasis*, DOI 10.1007/978-94-007-5678-6_8,

## Abbreviations

| | |
|---|---|
| EGF | epidermal growth factor |
| EGFR | epidermal growth factor receptor |
| IL | Interleukin |
| NK-cells | natural killer cells |
| Th1 | T-helper-1 |
| Th2 | T-helper-2 |
| VEGF | vascular endothelial growth factor |

## 8.1 Introduction

Cancer is one of the major causes of death in developed countries. While lung cancer is predominant in men (17%), women suffer most frequently from breast cancer (23%) (Jemal et al. 2011). The primary tumour itself can often be removed surgically, however, it is the subsequent development of metastases that is the leading cause of death in these patients: 90% of all cancer patients die from metastatic disease (Gupta and Massague 2006).

Intuitively one could assume that a compromised immune system in the perioperative period may play an important role in the genesis of metastases, since it theoretically leads to easier dissemination of malignant tumour cells released during surgery. Similarly, accelerated growth of pre-existing micrometastases may be the consequence of immune compromise in the perioperative setting (Ben-Eliyahu 2003). This impairment of immune function is considered to be multifactorial; anaesthetic and analgesic drugs are thought to play an integral role in this process. Hence, reducing the use of general anaesthetics and systemic analgesics and replacing these with regional anaesthetic and analgesic techniques may be a potential approach to a better outcome of patients undergoing cancer surgery.

This chapter discusses the present evidence on regional anaesthetic techniques and their assumed role in reducing the occurrence of postoperative metastases, thereby potentially influencing the outcome of patients.

## 8.2 Mechanism of Metastatic Disease

A balance between two conditions influences the development of metastases: Firstly, the metastatic potential of the original tumor and secondly the endogenous defence mechanisms of the patient (Snyder and Greenberg 2010). Initially, the primary tumor usually grows locally and its malignant cells are supplied with substrates by diffusion. With increasing tumor size angiogenic factors, synthesized by the tumour cells, lead to the formation of a distinct vascular and lymphatic supply and drain network. Subsequently, malignant cells invade this network and spread mainly through the lymphatic system. A large number of these cells are fended off through host defence mechanisms (Snyder and Greenberg 2010). However, those cells, that overcome host immune reactions, are potentially able to form micrometastases after extravasation in the capillary beds of distant organs (Fidler 2003). Natural killer cells (NK-cells) play a major role in the host defence mechanisms against tumour cells (Hashimoto et al. 2003). Their activity appears to be directly connected with the incidence of metastases. It has been shown that patients with a reduced activity of NK-cells also have an increased risk for cancer (Brittenden et al. 1996).

Some evidence exists that surgery itself may affect the incidence of metastases. One possible mechanism is a reduced NK-cell activity due to perioperative stress (Ben-Eliyahu et al. 1999). Other mechanisms that are currently discussed involve: (1) Direct tumour cell release into the circulation during surgery. (2) Discontinuation of secretion of angiogenesis inhibitors through the primary tumor after resection and subsequent increase of growth of latent micrometastases (Park et al. 2011, Snyder and Greenberg 2010). (3) Release of pro-angiogenesis factors, e.g. epidermal growth factor (EGF), prostaglandins E 1 and E 2 or vascular endothelial growth factor (VEGF) through manipulation during surgery (Snyder and Greenberg 2010).

On the other hand, anaesthesia itself may affect the development of metastases by direct effects of anaesthetics and systemic analgesics on immune function. Here discussion focuses on opioids which are thought to enhance the development of metastases. The suggested mechanism of promoting metastatic disease is mainly due to their immunosuppressive properties (Afsharimani et al. 2011).

Hence, reducing perioperative opioid consumption is currently discussed as an argument in favour of regional anaesthesia and its potentially inhibiting effects on the development of metastases. This chapter will discuss the impact of different types of regional anaesthetic techniques for tumour surgery on cancer re-occurrence based on the currently available evidence.

## 8.3 Effects of Local Anaesthetics

Regional anaesthesia/analgesia is provided by the injection or infusion of local anaesthetics. Local anaesthetics show a number of potentially beneficial effects in the setting of cancer surgery, as well with regard to direct inhibition of cancer cell proliferation as with regard to maintenance of immune function.

In a cancer model, lidocaine inhibits the epidermal growth factor receptor (EGFR) and thereby limits the proliferation of tongue cancer cells (Sakaguchi et al. 2006). The effect on EGF-mediated activities is also seen as the explanation for the reduction of invasiveness of cancer cells under the influence of lidocaine (Mammoto et al. 2002). Inhibitory effects on proliferation of cancer cells in vitro have also been shown for another local anaesthetic, ropivacaine (Martinsson 1999).

Furthermore, a recently published study showed a reduction of Interleukin (IL)-1 receptor antagonist and IL-6 in patients who received an intravenous infusion of lidocaine compared to a control group receiving saline. Simultaneously, the lymphocyte proliferation response to phytohemagglutinin-M was better maintained than in the placebo group (Yardeni et al. 2009). However, in the absence of surgery, local anaesthetics also abolish pain-induced increase in NK-cells activity and numbers (Greisen et al. 1999).

These findings suggest that local anaesthetics might lead to a reduced perioperative alteration of the immune system. However, the clinical significance of these promising systemic effects of local anaesthetics has not yet been confirmed.

## 8.4 Effect of Epidural Anaesthesia/Analgesia

It has been suggested that epidural analgesia reduces perioperative stress response, which might result in a better immune response of the patients (de Oliveira et al. 2011). It is obvious that the excellent analgesia provided by epidural techniques leads to an overall reduction of the requirement for other anaesthetic and analgesic agents in the perioperative period. However, evidence in this area remains controversial, in particular with regard to outcome data. A clinical benefit was found in some retrospective studies: In 2008, Biki and colleagues showed a considerable 57% decrease in the occurrence of metastases in patients undergoing surgery for prostate cancer and receiving a combined epidural and general anaesthesia compared to patients receiving general anaesthesia and a postoperative opioid based analgesia (Biki et al. 2008). However, limitations of this study should be considered when interpreting these results; First and foremost, this is a retrospective analysis which implies potential confounding factors. Furthermore, clinical and pharmacological methodological issues were subsequently raised due to missing details mainly on the epidural regimen, such as medications used and duration of analgesia (Daley and Norman 2009). A subsequent study found no evidence for a prolonged disease-free interval after radical prostatectomy with epidural analgesia (Tsui et al. 2010).

In another study, re-analysis of previous data showed a decrease in cancer recurrence in some patients undergoing colon surgery, when epidural analgesia was used (Christopherson et al. 2008). Patients in whom metastases at the time of surgery were not diagnosed, benefitted from an epidural analgesia within the first 1.46 years after surgery, while patients who received systemic opioid-based analgesia had a 4.65 times higher risk of dying ($p<0.012$). Later than 1.46 years post-surgery as well as in patients diagnosed with metastases at the time of surgery, no preventive effect of epidural analgesia was found.

Another recently published retrospective study did not find an association between the perioperative use of epidural analgesia and decreased cancer recurrence in patients undergoing colorectal cancer surgery (Gottschalk et al. 2010); only in a subgroup of patients over 64 years a slight benefit was detected.

As a further contribution to this topic, patients of the original "MASTER-trial" were assessed for cancer recurrence 9–15 years after surgery (Myles et al. 2011). Of the original 915 patients, 503 had surgery for cancer and of those 263 had been randomised to perioperative epidural analgesia and 240 patients to general anaesthesia with postoperative systemic opioids. The authors found that the recurrence-free interval in patients with and without epidural analgesia was not significantly different. The follow-up after 9–15 years was not planned at the design of the RCT, however this may be the only available randomised study available for years to come.

A very recently published retrospective study by Lai and colleagues suggested that any benefit of epidural analgesia on cancer recurrence may depend on the specific tumour type. They found in patients with small hepatocellular cancer undergoing percutaneous radiofrequency ablation a decrease in cancer recurrence, when general anaesthesia instead of epidural anaesthesia was performed (Lai et al. 2012).

This review of the literature demonstrates that despite an assumed conclusive mechanism, i.e. stress reduction and a consecutively improved perioperative immune function by epidural analgesia, clinical data remain contradictory. Taken together these data indicate that there is currently no evidence for a clinical beneficial effect of epidural analgesia on cancer recurrence. However, there is a significant lack of prospective data; well-designed prospective randomised trials in the future will probably provide more clarity on this topic and identify optimal treatment regimen for patients undergoing cancer surgery.

## 8.5 Paravertebral Block

Paravertebral blocks are an established alternative to epidural analgesia, in particular for unilateral thoracic surgery or combined with general anaesthesia for patients undergoing breast cancer surgery (Schnabel et al. 2010, Wenk and Schug 2011). A potential benefit aside from comparable analgesic efficacy to thoracic epidural analgesia is a potentially reduced adverse event profile (Wenk and Schug 2011).

Promising findings with regards to cancer recurrence were published by Exadaktylos and colleagues (2006). In a retrospective study in women undergoing breast cancer surgery they unveiled a reduced cancer recurrence when paravertebral block was combined with general anaesthesia in comparison to patients who received general anaesthesia and subsequent postoperative systemic analgesia. After 24 months the recurrence- and metastasis-free survival was 94% in the paravertebral group compared to 82% in the general anaesthesia group. At 36 months, this rate was 94% in the paravertebral compared to 77% in the general anaesthesia patients, respectively (Exadaktylos et al. 2006). However, these findings still need to be confirmed by prospective randomised controlled trials.

A currently ongoing, randomised multicenter trial, initiated by a group of investigators of the Cleveland Clinic is on the way to address these questions in a prospective manner; the group has published their study protocol in advance (Sessler et al. 2008). They will test the hypothesis that local or metastatic recurrence after breast cancer surgery is lower in patients randomized to paravertebral or high-thoracic epidural analgesia combined with sedation or light anaesthesia than in patients given intraoperative volatile anaesthesia and postoperative systemic opioid analgesia alone. According to the protocol the authors plan to enrol more than 1,100 patients with a follow-up period of at least 5 years. This is calculated to give 85% power for detecting a 30% treatment effect at an alpha of 0.05 (Sessler et al. 2008). Preliminary results of this investigation are expected soon.

Until then, potentially protective effects of paravertebral block with regard to cancer recurrence and occurrence of metastases must be regarded with caution. Paraverteral blocks for breast cancer surgery are conservatively used. New data on a potential positive effect in combination with a recently validated new approach to paravertebral catheter placement will hopefully lead to a more widespread use of this technique (Juttner et al. 2011).

## 8.6 Spinal Anaesthesia

To date, neither retrospective nor prospective clinical data exists evaluating the effect of spinal anaesthesia on cancer recurrence and metastatic disease. The underlying mechanism of a potentially protective effect mentioned above should probably be transferable to spinal anaesthesia, as suggested by animal data. In a rat model of laparotomy with tumour cell injection, one group of rats received general anaesthesia plus postoperative systemic opioids whereas the other group received general anaesthesia in combination with intrathecal bupivacaine and morphine. The incidence of metastases was decreased by the addition of spinal block (Bar-Yosef et al. 2001).

Another study found similar results in a mouse model; tumour immunity, including NK- and NKT-cell activity, was reduced after surgery when only inhalational general anaesthesia with perioperative systemic opioids was given instead of a balanced regimen with spinal anaesthesia (Wada et al. 2007). The cytokine balance between T-helper-1 (Th1) and T-helper-2 (Th2) was preserved.

The transferability of these findings onto human patients is questionable and has not been investigated to date. Considering that spinal anaesthesia can be regarded as self-contained technique, which does not necessarily need a top-up general anaesthesia, clinical data would be very interesting. Spinal anaesthesia ultimately offers the possibility to completely avoid any medication associated with a suppression of the immune system and potentially involved in the process of cancer recurrence and genesis of metastasis. The range of clinical use might include orthopaedic or dermatological tumour surgery of lower extremities. For using single shot spinal anaesthesia the intrathecal application of local anaesthetics such as bupivacaine can be combined with additives, like opioids or the central alpha-2-antagonist clonidine, to prolong the duration of effect. Efficacy and safety of these substances is well proved (Elia et al. 2008, Popping et al. 2012). A further alternative to single shot intrathecal anaesthesia might be the use of a continuous catheter-based spinal anaesthetic regimen.

## 8.7 Peripheral Nerve and Plexus Blocks

Peripheral nerve and plexus blocks have proven benefits in the control of peri- and postoperative pain (Popping et al. 2008), namely for surgical procedures of the upper and lower limbs. All blocks can be performed as a single shot or continuous catheter techniques. Medication used are mainly local anaesthetics, which can be supplemented by additives like central alpha-2-antagonists (Popping et al. 2009). It has been shown that the analgesic effect is superior compared to systemic opioids (Popping et al. 2008). Over the last few years, these peripheral regional anaesthetic techniques have gained popularity, mainly due to advances in ultrasound techniques and the introduction of affordable, portable and high-resolution ultrasound machines (Fingerman et al. 2009, Warman and Nicholls 2009). It is tempting to speculate that these techniques might have protective effects on cancer recurrence and incidence of metastatic disease in line with the mechanisms described above. Currently, however, there are no clinical data to support this hypothesis. One reason could be that surgical procedures for which these techniques are used are limited and major tumour surgery often involves thoracic or abdominal sites.

## 8.8 Conclusion

Basic pharmacological data on local anaesthetics and a number of in vitro and animal studies show the potential of regional anaesthesia to reduce recurrence of cancer and metastases. However, the clinical evidence for a potential protective effect of regional anaesthetic and analgesic techniques with respect to cancer recurrence and the incidence of metastases after tumour surgery is up to now inconclusive. Some retrospective studies show promising signs that epidural analgesia and paravertebral block may become stakeholders in this regard, but these need to be confirmed. Future prospective randomised controlled trials that address long-term outcomes may shed light on this topic. Furthermore, it is desirable that the range of regional anaesthetic techniques investigated in trials be wider and include techniques such as spinal anaesthesia and peripheral nerve blockade. Reassuringly, no effects of local anaesthetics or regional anaesthetic techniques are known to promote the growth of tumour or the development of metastases.

## References

Afsharimani B, Cabot P, Parat MO (2011) Morphine and tumor growth and metastasis. Cancer Metastasis Rev 30:225–238

Bar-Yosef S, Melamed R, Page GG, Shakhar G, Shakhar K, Ben-Eliyahu S (2001) Attenuation of the tumor-promoting effect of surgery by spinal blockade in rats. Anesthesiology 94:1066–1073

Ben-Eliyahu S (2003) The promotion of tumor metastasis by surgery and stress: immunological basis and implications for psychoneuroimmunology. Brain Behav Immun 17(Suppl 1):S27–36

Ben-Eliyahu S, Page GG, Yirmiya R, Shakhar G (1999) Evidence that stress and surgical interventions promote tumor development by suppressing natural killer cell activity. Int J Cancer 80:880–888

Biki B, Mascha E, Moriarty DC, Fitzpatrick JM, Sessler DI, Buggy DJ (2008) Anesthetic technique for radical prostatectomy surgery affects cancer recurrence: a retrospective analysis. Anesthesiology 109:180–187

Brittenden J, Heys SD, Ross J, Eremin O (1996) Natural killer cells and cancer. Cancer 77:1226–1243

Christopherson R, James KE, Tableman M, Marshall P, Johnson FE (2008) Long-term survival after colon cancer surgery: a variation associated with choice of anesthesia. Anesth Analg 107:325–332

Daley MD, Norman PH (2009) Retrospective but not rigorous. Anesthesiology 111:203 (author reply 203–204)

de Oliveira GS, Jr AS, Schink JC, Singh DK, Fitzgerald PC, McCarthy RJ (2011) Intraoperative neuraxial anesthesia but not postoperative neuraxial analgesia is associated with increased relapse-free survival in ovarian cancer patients after primary cytoreductive surgery. Reg Anesth Pain Med 36:271–277

Elia N, Culebras X, Mazza C, Schiffer E, Tramer MR (2008) Clonidine as an adjuvant to intrathecal local anesthetics for surgery: systematic review of randomized trials. Reg Anesth Pain Med 33:159–167

Exadaktylos AK, Buggy DJ, Moriarty DC, Mascha E, Sessler DI (2006) Can anesthetic technique for primary breast cancer surgery affect recurrence or metastasis? Anesthesiology 105:660–664

Fidler IJ (2003) The pathogenesis of cancer metastasis: the 'seed and soil' hypothesis revisited. Nat Rev Cancer 3:453–458

Fingerman M, Benonis JG, Martin G (2009) A practical guide to commonly performed ultrasound-guided peripheral-nerve blocks. Curr Opin Anaesthesiol 22:600–607

Gottschalk A, Ford JG, Regelin CC, You J, Mascha EJ, Sessler DI, Durieux ME, Nemergut EC (2010) Association between epidural analgesia and cancer recurrence after colorectal cancer surgery. Anesthesiology 113:27–34

Greisen J, Hokland M, Grofte T, Hansen PO, Jensen TS, Vilstrup H, Tonnesen E (1999) Acute pain induces an instant increase in natural killer cell cytotoxicity in humans and this response is abolished by local anaesthesia. Br J Anaesth 83:235–240

Gupta GP, Massague J (2006) Cancer metastasis: building a framework. Cell 127:679–695

Hashimoto W, Tanaka F, Robbins PD, Taniguchi M, Okamura H, Lotze MT, Tahara H (2003) Natural killer, but not natural killer T, cells play a necessary role in the promotion of an innate antitumor response induced by IL-18. Int J Cancer 103:508–513

Jemal A, Bray F, Center MM, Ferlay J, Ward E, Forman D (2011) Global cancer statistics. CA Cancer J Clin 61:69–90

Juttner T, Werdehausen R, Hermanns H, Monaca E, Danzeisen O, Pannen BH, Janni W, Winterhalter M (2011) The paravertebral lamina technique: a new regional anesthesia approach for breast surgery. J Clin Anesth 23:443–450

Lai R, Peng Z, Chen D, Wang X, Xing W, Zeng W, Chen M (2012) The effects of anesthetic technique on cancer recurrence in percutaneous radiofrequency ablation of small hepatocellular carcinoma. Anesth Analg 114:290–296

Mammoto T, Higashiyama S, Mukai M, Mammoto A, Ayaki M, Mashimo T, Hayashi Y, Kishi Y, Nakamura H, Akedo H (2002) Infiltration anesthetic lidocaine inhibits cancer cell invasion by modulating ectodomain shedding of heparin-binding epidermal growth factor-like growth factor (HB-EGF). J Cell Physiol 192:351–358

Martinsson T (1999) Ropivacaine inhibits serum-induced proliferation of colon adenocarcinoma cells in vitro. J Pharmacol Exp Ther 288:660–664

Myles PS, Peyton P, Silbert B, Hunt J, Rigg JR, Sessler DI, Trials Group Investigators ANZCA (2011) Perioperative epidural analgesia for major abdominal surgery for cancer and recurrence-free survival: randomised trial. BMJ 342:d1491

Park Y, Kitahara T, Takagi R, Kato R (2011) Does surgery for breast cancer induce angiogenesis and thus promote metastasis? Oncology 81:199–205

Popping DM, Zahn PK, Van Aken HK, Dasch B, Boche R, Pogatzki-Zahn EM (2008) Effectiveness and safety of postoperative pain management: a survey of 18 925 consecutive patients between 1998 and 2006 (2nd revision): a database analysis of prospectively raised data. Br J Anaesth 101:832–840

Popping DM, Elia N, Marret E, Wenk M, Tramer MR (2009) Clonidine as an adjuvant to local anesthetics for peripheral nerve and plexus blocks: a meta-analysis of randomized trials. Anesthesiology 111:406–415

Popping DM, Elia N, Marret E, Wenk M, Tramer MR (2012) Opioids added to local anesthetics for single-shot intrathecal anesthesia in patients undergoing minor surgery: a meta-analysis of randomized trials. Pain 153(4):784–93

Sakaguchi M, Kuroda Y, Hirose M (2006) The antiproliferative effect of lidocaine on human tongue cancer cells with inhibition of the activity of epidermal growth factor receptor. Anesth Analg 102:1103–1107

Schnabel A, Reichl SU, Kranke P, Pogatzki-Zahn EM, Zahn PK (2010) Efficacy and safety of paravertebral blocks in breast surgery: a meta-analysis of randomized controlled trials. Br J Anaesth 105:842–852

Sessler DI, Ben-Eliyahu S, Mascha EJ, Parat MO, Buggy DJ (2008) Can regional analgesia reduce the risk of recurrence after breast cancer? Methodology of a multicenter randomized trial. Contemp Clin Trials 29:517–526

Snyder GL, Greenberg S (2010) Effect of anaesthetic technique and other perioperative factors on cancer recurrence. Br J Anaesth 105:106–115

Tsui BC, Rashiq S, Schopflocher D, Murtha A, Broemling S, Pillay J, Finucane BT (2010) Epidural anesthesia and cancer recurrence rates after radical prostatectomy. Can J Anaesth 57:107–112

Wada H, Seki S, Takahashi T, Kawarabayashi N, Higuchi H, Habu Y, Sugahara S, Kazama T (2007) Combined spinal and general anesthesia attenuates liver metastasis by preserving TH1/TH2 cytokine balance. Anesthesiology 106:499–506

Warman P, Nicholls B (2009) Ultrasound-guided nerve blocks: efficacy and safety. Best Pract Res Clin Anaesthesiol 23:313–326

Wenk M, Schug SA (2011) Perioperative pain management after thoracotomy. Curr Opin Anaesthesiol 24:8–12

Yardeni IZ, Beilin B, Mayburd E, Levinson Y, Bessler H (2009) The effect of perioperative intravenous lidocaine on postoperative pain and immune function. Anesth Analg 109:1464–1469

# Chapter 9
# Perioperative Morphine and Cancer Recurrence

**Ashley M. Shilling and Mohamed Tiouririne**

**Abstract** There is growing evidence suggesting that certain interventions during the perioperative period may have an impact on long-term outcomes of patients undergoing cancer surgery. It has been postulated that regional anesthetic techniques and other targeted interventions could decrease the risk of cancer recurrence, therefore increasing the disease-free interval and overall survival, of those patients undergoing cancer surgery. Conversely, however, it has also been theorized that volatile anesthetics, opioids and surgery itself are directly or indirectly linked to cancer recurrence. Among the opioids used during the perioperative period, morphine has raised most of the concerns regarding its putative effects on cancer. Indeed, morphine has been found to affect many cellular and cell signaling pathways involved in cancer genesis and possibly causing tumor growth. This chapter will focus on the role of the perioperative period on cancer progression, the recognized mechanisms of action of morphine on cancer and alternative pain management options for patients undergoing cancer surgery.

**Keywords** Analgesia • Anesthesia • Cancer • Morphine • Metastasis • Opioids • Pain management • Surgery

A.M. Shilling, M.D.
Associate Professor of Anesthesiology and Obstetric and Gynecology, University of Virginia, PO BOX 800710, Charlottesville, VA 22908, USA
e-mail: abm5f@virginia.edu

M. Tiouririne, M.D. (✉)
Department of Anesthesiology and Obstetrics and Gynecology, University of Virginia, PO BOX 800710, Charlottesville, VA 22908, USA
e-mail: mt9y@virginia.edu

M.-O. Parat (ed.), *Morphine and Metastasis*, DOI 10.1007/978-94-007-5678-6_9, 

## Abbreviations

| | |
|---|---|
| cAMP | cyclic adenosine monophosphate |
| COX-2 | cyclooxygenase 2 |
| HIF | hypoxia inducible transcription factor |
| NK | natural killer |
| NO | nitric oxide |
| NSAIDs | non-steroidal anti-inflammatory drugs |
| PMN | polymorphonuclear leucocyte |
| PGE2 | prostaglandin E2 |
| STAT-3 | signal transducer of activation and transcription-3 |
| VEGF | vascular endothelial growth factor |

## 9.1 Introduction

Morphine, the naturally occurring alkaloid extracted of the milky juice of the poppy plant "opium", was first extracted by the German pharmacist, *Frederich W. Serturner* in 1806. He derived its name from the Greek god of dream, "*Morpheus*" for its stupor-like effects. However, the history of its use can be traced all the way back to the third millennium BC (Stein and Rosow 2004) in ancient Iraq. Merck was first to commercialize morphine in 1827. Following the discovery of the hypodermic needle in 1857, morphine began being utilized as a sedative in anesthesiology practice and also to alleviate pain following surgical procedures. To date, morphine is still referred to as the prototypal analgesic to which all other opioids are compared, and it is the most commonly used analgesic during the perioperative stage. Over the years, morphine has received a favorable safety profile though it still has several well known short-term side effects among which, respiratory depression and constipation are the most troublesome. However, in recent years, there have been concerns in the literature over the role of morphine in tumor recurrence and metastasis following cancer surgery. Consequently, this long-term effect of morphine has caused its relevance in the perioperative period as the analgesic of choice for patients undergoing cancer surgery to be controversial (Afsharimani et al. 2011). The tumor-enhancing effects of morphine seem to result from the fact that opioids and morphine in particular alter immune function (Sacerdote 2008), the first line of defense against cancer; stimulate angiogenesis (Pasi et al. 1991) and enhance vascular permeability (Moss and Rosow 2008), which represents an impetus to tumor metastasis. Despite these facts, it would be naïve to consider that morphine is the only party responsible for tumor recurrence and metastasis following cancer surgery. The determinants of cancer recurrence following surgery have been attributed to many factors. These include the surgical stress response (Ben-Eliyahu 2003), inflammatory response (Salo 1996), anesthetic choices (Snyder and Greenberg 2010), minimal residual disease (Goldfarb and Ben-Eliyahu 2006), escape from dormancy (Demicheli et al. 2005), the surgery itself (Ben-Eliyahu 2003) and ultimately opioid choice (Afsharimani et al. 2011).

## 9.2 The Perioperative Period and Cancer Recurrence

Surgery is undeniably an integral component of the management of many solid tumors and cancer in general. However, it is also recognized that surgery may promote local recurrence and distant metastasis. The negative impact of surgical manipulation on cancer recurrence and progression were known for millennia. A. Cornelius Celsus was first to recognize that only encapsulated tumors should be removed because the other stages would be irritated and exacerbated by surgery. Likewise, Alfred Velpeau (1795–1867) observed that operations for cancer were correlated with the return of the disease and tended to accelerate tumor growth (Raven 1990). To translate these earlier observations to modern medicine, many theories have been advanced. In addition to tumor manipulation, which releases free cancer cells in the bloodstream with a potential for distant seeding (Yamashita et al. 2000), surgery itself provokes profound metabolic, neuroendocrine, immunologic and inflammatory derangements. These latter derangements could also be the trigger for tumor homeostasis breakdown during the perioperative period. The depression of the immune system following surgery has also been implicated in the development of recurrence (Page 2005). Finally, escape from dormancy, whereby deregulation in the equilibrium between activators and inhibitors of angiogenesis imposed by surgery, could hypothetically set off the "angiogenic switch" and therefore recurrence.

### *9.2.1 Surgery and Inflammatory Response*

The impact of surgery on various organ systems has been termed "*systemic response to surgery or surgical stress response*". This stress response stimulates release of pro-inflammatory cytokines (IL-1; IL-6; TNF; PAF) that have been directly or indirectly implicated in cancer genesis. The inflammatory response to surgery or the acute-phase reactant, results in a cascade of chain reactions leading to cytokine release. In particular, IL-6 and IL-1β have been shown to upregulate the expression of vascular endothelial growth factor (VEGF). McMillan et al., have shown that persistent acute-phase response was associated with a higher rate of relapse after curative surgery for colon cancer (McMillan et al. 1995). Recently, in a mouse model, a high level of cytokines (IL-1 and IL-1β) was associated with increased angiogenesis and tumor growth following laparotomy (Pera et al. 2003). The hypothesis that the perioperative acute phase reactant might be linked to cancer recurrence lies in the similarity of various pro-inflammatory mediators with those produced by the tumor microenvironment. This tumor microenvironment or tumor stroma represents the force by which tumor cells acquire nutrients for growth, gain new blood vessels, start the invasion process, and ultimately attain metastatic potential (Marx 2008). In this stroma lies a sophisticated organization of malignant pathways where several mediators of the inflammatory response have influence. Therefore, surgery and inflammatory response could potentially upregulate the factors in the tumor microenvironment fueling tumor growth (Fig. 9.1).

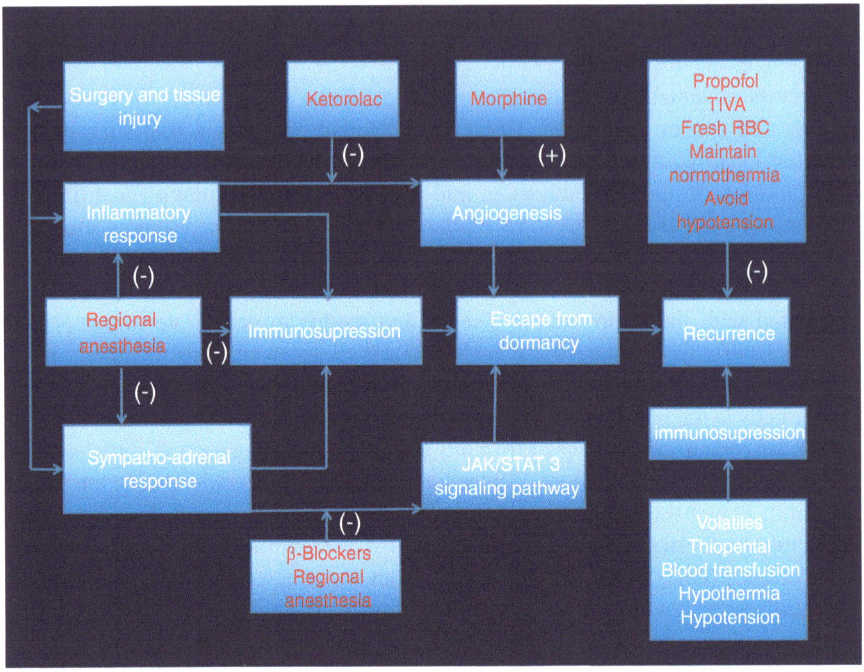


**Fig. 9.1** Perioperative factors involved in cancer recurrence. *TIVA* total intravenous anesthesia, *RBC* red blood cells. (+) possible negative effect: more recurrence, (-) possible positive effect: less recurrence

## 9.2.2 Surgery and the Immune System

Surgery and surgical trauma stimulate major physiological changes on human body homeostasis. The immune system appears to be affected as well. It has been shown that surgery affects the immune system for several days postoperatively and this correlated well with the invasiveness of the surgery (Page 2005). One theory that might explain the effect of surgery on the immune system resides in the fact that, at the time of surgery, opposing inflammatory sequences regulate the immune response to surgical and tissue trauma. These two opposing physiological events act to maintain a balance of the immune system and are part of the overall surgical inflammatory response. First, the acute phase reactant or pro-inflammatory phase involves cells of the innate immune system. Second, the compensatory anti-inflammatory response phase is regulated by the cells of the adaptive immune system. It is postulated that an uncoupling of the pro-inflammatory-anti-inflammatory balance could be responsible for the immune suppression seen after surgery (Bone 1996; Faist et al. 1996). Additionally, the neuro-sympatho-endocrine system plays an important role in perioperative immunosupression; this is due to the release of catecholamines and glucocorticoids during the surgical trauma (Kurosawa and Kato 2008; Reiche et al. 2004). Moreover, glucocorticoids are known immune-suppressants (Keh et al. 2003); their secretion in abundance in the perioperative period is partially responsible for the weakening of the immune function following surgery. Likewise, the catecholamines norepinephrine and epinephrine are also responsible for the depression of the immune system, most notably cellular mediated immunity, and affect cell migration and invasiveness. This appears to be related to the activation of β-receptors and cyclic adenosine monophosphate (cAMP) production (Masur et al. 2001; Thaker et al. 2006; Yang et al. 2006). However, catecholamines have also been implicated in cancer genesis via other mechanisms such as the stimulation of the STAT-3 (signal transducer of activation and transcription) pathway (Landen et al. 2007) or VEGF production (Lutgendorf et al. 2003).

## 9.3 Mechanisms of Action of Morphine on Cancer

In recent years, morphine has been the center of many discussions regarding its implication in cancer growth. Indeed several reports suggest that the effects of morphine on the immune system, angiogenesis and apoptosis could be responsible for such observations. However, this should be counterbalanced by other observations of morphine's tumoricidal effects. Although the use of morphine during the perioperative period could singly contribute to cancer metastasis and recurrence, it is probable that this effect is multifactorial (Table 9.1).

### *9.3.1 Immune Function*

It is well known that pain causes immune suppression, and its treatment is therefore very important. However, it has also been established that opioids cause inhibition of both cellular and humoral immune function (Sacerdote 2008). Human clinical data implicating morphine as a direct impetus for cancer recurrence is lacking, however in-vivo and in-vitro experiments suggest that possibility. The relationship between the immune system and morphine in particular has raised many questions regarding opioid use in certain patient populations. Indeed, in patients with an already compromised immune system such as those with malignancies, an additional suppression may ultimately be detrimental. During the early stage of malignancies, cancerous cells are recognized as non-self and therefore exposed to the effect of natural killer (NK) cytotoxic activity and activated T cells and other modulators of the immune system. During the phases of immuno-editing, a three step process by which cancer cells are handled by the immune system, cancer cells constantly change their antigenic make up. This results in the ability of subsets of cancer cells to evade the immune system and become overt tumors (Dunn et al. 2004). It is therefore postulated that when the immune system is already depressed, such as during the perioperative period, morphine exposure could accelerate this process

**Table 9.1** Overview of reported effects of anesthetic, analgesic and other perioperative factors on cancer progression

| |
|---|
| **Surgical stress response and cancer** |
| Stress and surgical excision of the primary tumor can promote tumor metastasis (Ben-Eliyahu 2003; Melamed et al. 2005) |
| **Neuroendocrine system** |
| General anesthesia accompanied by surgical stress may suppress immunity, presumably by directly affecting the immune system or activating the hypothalamic-pituitary-adrenal axis and the sympathetic nervous system (Kurosawa and Kato 2008) |
| **Inflammatory system** |
| Promotion of cancer progression, through immunosupression via cytokines, chemokines, prostaglandins, cyclooxygenase (Kundu and Surh 2008) |
| **Pain** |
| Suppression of NK-cell activity (Sacerdote et al. 1994; Shavit et al. 1987) and promotion of tumor development in animals (Lewis et al. 1983) |
| **Opiates** |
| Opioids inhibit cellular and humoral immune function in humans (Sacerdote et al. 2000). Morphine inhibits spontaneous and cytokine-enhanced natural killer cell cytotoxicity (Yeager et al. 1995; Beilin et al. 1989). *In contrast:* Intravenous fentanyl increases natural killer cell cytotoxicity and circulating CD16 (+) lymphocytes in humans (Yeager et al. 2002) |
| Opioid- induced promotion and stimulation of angiogenesis (Gupta et al. 2002) |
| **Beta-adrenergic blockade** |
| β-Blocker (nadolol) and a prostaglandin synthesis inhibitor (indomethacin), attenuated the metastasis-promoting effects of surgery when used alone or in combination (Melamed et al. 2005) |
| **Cyclooxygenase inhibitors** |
| COX inhibitors may prevent metastatic progression and attenuate opiate-induced immunosuppression in rats (Melamed et al. 2005). The combination of COX-2 inhibitor etodolac and ß-blocker propanolol can efficiently prevent immunosuppression following surgery (Benish et al. 2008). COX-2 inhibitor celecoxib prevents chronic morphine-induced promotion of angiogenesis, tumour growth, metastasis and mortality in a murine breast cancer model (Farooqui et al. 2007) |
| **Anesthetic induction agents and volatile anesthetics** |
| Suppression of natural killer cell activity and promotion of tumor metastasis by ketamine, thiopental, and halothane (Melamed et al. 2005) |
| **Regional anesthesia** |
| Studies in animals show that regional anesthesia and optimal postoperative analgesia independently reduce metastasis (Wada et al. 2007; Bar-Yosef et al. 2001). Retrospective studies in humans support a benefit of regional analgesia for patients undergoing surgery for breast, colon and prostate cancer with respect to reduction of recurrence (Exadaktylos et al. 2006; Biki et al. 2008; Christopherson et al. 2008) |
| **Perioperative blood transfusion** |
| Perioperative blood transfusion is associated with poorer outcome for patients with colorectal cancer recurrence (Amato and Pescatori 2006) |
| **Perioperative hypothermia** |
| Hypothermia leads to a reduction in cell-mediated immunity, particularly NK-cells, and an increase in lung tumor retention and metastasis in rats (Ben-Eliyahu et al. 1999) |

Reprinted with permission Gottschalk et al. (2010b, 110(6): 1638)

of immunosupression and ultimately favor recurrence (Gottschalk et al. 2010a). Morphine exerts it effects through inhibition of many components of the immune system. These include phagocytic activity (Vallejo et al. 2004), cytolytic T lymphocyte activity (Mellon and Bayer 1998) and NK cell activity (Beilin et al. 1989, 1996). The actions of morphine on the immune cells are probably mediated through the μ opioid receptor, but also via interaction with the hypothalamic-pituitary-adrenal (HPA) axis. However, morphine was also found to have protective effects towards tumors. This potentially beneficial effect of morphine was attributed to enhanced T cell-mediated response (Fuggetta et al. 2005), a splice variant of μ opioid receptor (Cadet et al. 2003), inhibition of the nuclear factor κB (Sueoka et al. 1998) and activation of the nitric oxide synthase pathway (Welters et al. 2000).

### 9.3.2 Angiogenesis

The effects of morphine on angiogenesis are complex and are beyond the scope of this chapter, they are discussed in more details elsewhere in this book. Angiogenesis, the formation of new vessels, represents a sine qua non condition for tumor development, proliferation and invasion. In several in-vitro and in-vivo models of tumor and non-tumor cell growth, morphine was found to promote angiogenesis. Indeed, μ opioid receptors are found on the surface of endothelial cells and they increase the release of intracellular calcium and nitric oxide (NO). The release of NO mediates vascular permeability, endothelial cell proliferation, migration and ultimately angiogenesis. It seems that this effect is in part due to NO-dependent MAPK phosphorylation and endothelial growth (Leo et al. 2009). Additionally, it was postulated that morphine upregulates cyclooxygenase 2 (COX-2), and Prostaglandin E2 (PGE2), known to be angiogenic factors. Farooqui et al. demonstrated that co-administration of Celecoxib, a COX-2 inhibitor, prevented morphine stimulation of COX-2 and PGE2, angiogenesis, tumor growth, metastasis, and mortality in a murine breast cancer model (Farooqui et al. 2007). In contradiction, however, morphine has been found to be anti-angiogenic. Using Lewis lung carcinoma cells, Koodie et al. found that morphine inhibited hypoxia inducible transcription factors (HIF) (Koodie et al. 2010). HIF are transcription factors that modulate several genes to promote survival during hypoxic conditions including vascular endothelial growth factor (VEGF).

### 9.3.3 Apoptosis

Apoptosis, also termed programmed cell death, is an important step in maintaining physiological body equilibrium. This programmed cell death is mediated via caspase 3 and the Bcl-2 pathways (Kelly and Strasser 2011). Undoubtedly, this process is inhibited when normal cells acquire malignant potential, resulting in tumor growth and proliferation (Hanahan and Weinberg 2000; Hengartner 2000). It has been shown in several models of cancer cells that morphine exerts both pro-apoptotic and anti-apoptotic effects. The effects of morphine on apoptosis were described by Yin and al on freshly isolated peripheral blood lymphocytes (Yin et al. 1999). Equally, in lung cancer cells, Yoshida et al. demonstrated the apoptotic properties of opioids analgesics (Yoshida et al. 2000). Additionally, fentanyl, a common opioid analgesic, was found to have apoptotic effects as well (Delogu et al. 2004). Several other studies have consistently reported the pro-apoptotic effects of morphine on both tumor and non-tumor cells. These effects of morphine are mediated through a μ opioid (Gupta et al. 2002) and non-opioid receptor-dependent mechanisms (Lin et al. 2009; Tegeder et al. 2003). Conflicting with its pro-apoptotic effects, morphine has also been shown to be anti-apoptotic (Iglesias et al. 2003) and therefore could potentially promote tumor growth. The combined effect of anti-apoptosis, promotion of angiogenesis and immunosupression has led to the discussion of morphine deleterious effect on cancer progression during the perioperative period.

## 9.4 Alternative Strategies to Pain Management

With growing interest in the use of narcotics during the perioperative period, with greatest focus on morphine, and cancer progression, alternative pain management strategies as well as approaches to anesthesia in patient undergoing cancer surgery have been proposed. Thus, the use of epidural analgesia and opioid-sparing anesthetic techniques have emerged as potential approaches for reducing recurrences following cancer surgery.

### *9.4.1 Local Anesthetics*

Local anesthetics have been in clinical use for more than a century and during this time, their application has expanded exponentially. Common clinical uses include topical, infiltration, field block, neuraxial and peripheral nerve block techniques as well as continuous infusions. Local anesthetics exert their major mechanism of action on the alpha subunit of sodium channels. While sodium channels are located throughout the body, the intended analgesic target of local anesthetics is neural tissue with subsequent blockade of impulse conduction. The result is a sensory and motor blockade; a feature which lends itself nicely to perioperative analgesia and anesthesia. In addition to blockade of sodium channels, local anesthetics have been shown to affect many other systems. Of particular interest, local anesthetics can exert effects on inflammatory cells and mediators as well as other cells including erythrocytes and thrombocytes. Because malignant disease states and surgeries impose a significant stress on the body, the anti-inflammatory properties of local anesthetics may significantly affect the response of the body to these stressors and the resultant inflammatory state and immune response. There is widespread speculation that these effects of local anesthetics could offer protection against malignancies and malignant metastasis in the perioperative period. Additionally, the resulting decrease in cellular immunity and pro-angiogenic factors induced by the tissue trauma of surgery may be offset or even inhibited by local anesthetics. In vitro and in vivo, local anesthetics have been shown to exert a multitude of effects on the inflammatory system. They may lead to attenuation or a decrease in neurogenic inflammation (Coderre et al. 1993). Local anesthetics also have inherent anti-inflammatory properties, which may directly affect the inflammatory response. Through inhibition of leukocyte functions, local anesthetics impact the human response to tissue trauma or stress. Firstly, local anesthetics inhibit leukocyte adhesion (Azuma et al. 2000; Schmidt et al. 1997). This is true for local anesthetic doses commonly used in clinical practice (MacGregor et al. 1980). The mechanism by which local anesthetics affect adhesion is thought to be multi-factorial and includes their effect on integrins and leukocyte adhesion molecule-1 (Cassuto et al. 2006). In addition to adhesion, local anesthetics also inhibit polymorphonuclear leukocyte (PMN) migration through several proposed mechanisms (Hollmann et al. 2001; Mikawa et al. 2003). In addition to their direct effects on leukocytes, Local anesthetics also affect other mediators of inflammation including prostaglandins, histamine, cytokines, and leukotrienes. Local anesthetics have been demonstrated to block leukotriene release from PMNs and monocytes as well as interleukin-1 alpha release from peripheral blood mononuclear cells (Sinclair et al. 1993). Additionally, lidocaine inhibits histamine release from basophils and mast cells (Yanagi et al. 1996). The importance of these actions in the realm of cancer progression is still to be determined.

In addition to their anti-inflammatory actions, local anesthetics stimulate the activity of NK cells in the perioperative setting, thus leading to important changes and consequences in the cancer patient. NK cells are derived from bone marrow and are an important component of non-specific cellular-mediated and antitumor immunity. NK cells possess the ability to lyse tumors both in vitro and in vivo without the need for prior sensitization. Patients with lower levels of NK cells have been shown to have a higher incidence of cancers (Brittenden et al. 1996). NK cells have been shown to eliminate metastatic cells in the circulation and are even considered to be the primary defense against cancers (Anderson 2005). Thus, the role of NK cells in tumor formation and metastasis is one that has created significant interest in cancer research. In the 1980s, scientists began looking at NK cells as a means of treating patients with high tumor burden or metastasis (Rosenberg et al. 1993). Since that time, there have been numerous studies using NK cells in hopes of affecting cancer progression and recurrence. While it has been shown that many pharmacologic agents used in the peri-operative period have negative effects on NK cells and thus, might worsen cancer outcomes, local anesthetics may actually have a positive effect on NK cells. Forget et al. performed a systematic review of the literature on NK activity during the perioperative period and found that local anesthetics, contrary to opioids and most other anesthetics, actually stimulate the activity of NK cells (Forget and De Kock 2009).

There are marked changes of immune response immediately following surgery, and the immune system and stress response can be affected for as long as 3–4 days post-operatively (Christopherson et al. 1993). Therefore, this may be a crucial time in which minimal residual disease may grow and metastasize. Thus, this period may be a critical window in which specific factors could affect longer-term prognosis including the host immune response to cancerous cells and the likelihood of metastasis. With our growing understanding of the effects of local anesthetics on immunomodulation and inflammation, interest has shifted to human studies and the clinical setting. Yardeni et al. assessed pain intensity and immune reactivity in two groups of female patients undergoing trans-abdominal surgery receiving either intravenous lidocaine started 20 min before surgery, or a placebo. All patients received patient-controlled epidural analgesia. In the intravenous lidocaine group, not only were pain scores improved, but also, production of pro-inflammatory cytokines IL-1ra and IL-6 were significantly reduced. This study indicates that intravenous lidocaine reduces surgery-induced immune alterations, potentially affecting cancer recurrence (Yardeni et al. 2009). Likewise, Hong et al. studied a cohort of women undergoing laparoscopic radical hysterectomy for cervical cancer and demonstrated a reduction in IL-6 levels and an earlier normalization of IL-2 in patients who received preemptive lidocaine and morphine as compared with those who received an epidural without any preemptive treatment (Hong and Lim 2008). It appears that the use of intravenous lidocaine could hypothetically offset some of the effects of morphine when the two drugs are used in combination.

### *9.4.2 Regional Anesthesia*

The use of epidurals and peripheral nerve block procedures has been shown to affect markers of immunomodulation and inflammation. Data suggests that epidural anesthesia may completely block the sympathetic response to surgery below the umbilicus and blunt the response above the umbilicus (Kehlet 1989; Magnusdottir et al. 1999). Animal studies have demonstrated some positive effects of neuraxially-administered local anesthetics on the inflammatory response, NK cells, and the potential to affect cancer recurrence. In a rat model, Bar-Yosef et al. demonstrated that the addition of a spinal anesthetic to an inhalational anesthesia with halothane attenuated the promotion of metastasis after pulmonary tumor cells were injected (Bar-Yosef et al. 2001). In another rodent model, the addition of a spinal anesthetic to sevoflurane anesthesia significantly decreased the number of liver metastases. The authors speculated that this was due to the effects of local anesthetic on cytokines (Wada et al. 2007).

With encouraging results on the potential for regional anesthetic techniques to influence patient stress response to surgery, focus has shifted to patients undergoing procedures for malignancy and outcomes related to their cancers. Studies have examined the delivery of local anesthetics through various mechanisms including local infiltration, neuraxial administration (epidural or spinal), or through peripheral approaches such as a paravertebral block. Schlagenhauff et al. conducted one of the first published studies that sparked significant interest in the question of whether the modality of anesthesia affects cancer-related outcomes (Schlagenhauff et al. 2000).

This group retrospectively examined more than 4,000 patients undergoing melanoma excision with either general anesthesia or local anesthesia. The patients who underwent general anesthesia had a decrease in survival with a relative risk of 1.46. Another retrospective study of 129 women undergoing breast cancer surgery was performed by Exadaktylos et al. The anesthetic regimen entailed either a general anesthetic with morphine or a general anesthetic with a paravertebral block using a local anesthetic (Exadaktylos et al. 2006). The authors found that patients who received a paravertebral block had a significantly higher metastasis-free period in the first 36 months after surgery as compared to the patients who underwent general anesthesia without a block (82 % survival vs. 77 %). In a retrospective study, Biki et al. similarly examined patients with prostate cancer. They demonstrated the association of a regional technique with a lower incidence of biochemical recurrence of prostate cancer in 225 patients undergoing radical prostatectomy surgery. Both groups of patients received a general anesthetic but they received either an epidural for analgesia, or post-operative opioids. In a 10-year follow-up, the relative risk reduction was 57 % in patients that received an epidural in addition to their general anesthetic (Biki et al. 2008). Despite the initial encouraging results demonstrating reduced recurrence and improved survival in patients receiving adjuvant local anesthetics and regional techniques, a number of studies have shown discouraging results. Three additional studies examining malignancy recurrence in prostate cancer showed no significant differences in cancer recurrence in patient receiving general anesthesia with or without an epidural. In a secondary analysis of a randomized controlled trial, Tsui et al. did not find a difference in biochemical markers among patients who received epidural analgesia vs. general anesthesia (Tsui et al. 2010). Likewise, Wuethrich et al. did not find a difference in biochemical markers of recurrence of prostate cancer; however, they noted an improvement in clinical progression-free interval in the epidural group (Wuethrich et al. 2011). Furthermore, Forget at al. were unable to demonstrate improved outcomes with the use of epidural as compared to other conventional pain control modalities and other pain control modalities in their retrospective review of 1,111 consecutives prostate surgeries. However the authors noted that the use of sufentanil, a synthetic opioid, was associated with an increase risk of relapse (Forget et al. 2010). Of note, Myles et al. published the results of a randomized controlled trial comparing general anesthesia with opioids to general anesthesia with epidural analgesia in patients undergoing various abdominal surgeries. Although the primary outcome was not cancer recurrence, in a subset of patients who did undergo cancer surgery, the investigators did not demonstrate any benefit of epidural analgesia with respect to cancer recurrence (Myles et al. 2011).

Other promising retrospective analyses comparing intraoperative epidural to general anesthesia were published thereafter with conflicting results (Table 9.2). In conclusion, it appears that the use of epidural analgesia in conjunction with general anesthesia could potentially improve outcomes in patients undergoing cancer surgery. Additionally, local anesthetics appear to offer a multitude of effects, which could also lead to outcome improvements in the cancer patient. However, we are far from a consensus regarding the widespread use of epidural analgesia for this indication

**Table 9.2** Clinical studies comparing the effect of different modes of anesthesia and analgesia on cancer recurrence or metastasis

| Authors | Study type | Type of cancer | Anesthetic | Outcomes |
|---|---|---|---|---|
| Seebacher et al. (1990) | Retrospective | Melanoma | GA<br>LA | Inconclusive |
| Melchi et al. (1995) | Retrospective | Melanoma | GA<br>Neuroleptanalgesia vs. LA | Favors LA |
| Schlagenhauf et al. (1995) | Retrospective | Melanoma | GA<br>LA | Favors LA |
| Exadaktylos et al. (2006) | Retrospective | Breast | GA + PVA<br>GA + PCA | Favors PVA |
| Biki et al. (2008) | Retrospective | Prostate | GA + EA<br>GA + PCA | Favors EA |
| Christopherson et al. (2008) | Prospective | Colon | GA + EA<br>GA + IV [MSO4] | Favors EA[a] |
| Tsui et al. (2010) | Retrospective | Prostate | GA + EA<br>GA + IV [MSO4] | No difference |
| Forget et al. (2010) | Retrospective | Breast | Sufentanil, ketamine, NSAIDs, clonidine. | Favors NSAIDs [Ketorolac] |
| Lin et al. (2011) | Retrospective | Ovarian | GA + EA<br>GA + IV [MSO4] | Favors EA |
| Gottschalk et al. (2010 b) | Retrospective | Colon | GA + EA<br>GA + IV opioids | Favors EA[b] |
| Fleischmann et al. (2009) | Prospective | Colon | GA without $NO_2$<br>GA with $NO_2$ | No difference |
| Ismail et al. (2010) | Retrospective | Cervical | GA<br>Neuraxial | No difference |
| Myles et al. (2011) | Prospective | Various abdominal cancers | GA + EA<br>GA + PCA [MSO4] | No difference |

| | | | | |
|---|---|---|---|---|
| Oliveira et al. (2011) | Retrospective | Ovarian | GA + EA<br>GA + EA [Post-op]<br>GA + PCA [MSO4] | Favors EA[c] |
| Gupta et al. (2011) | Retrospective | Colo-rectal | GA + EA<br>GA + PCA [MSO4] | Favors EA[d] |
| Forget et al. (2011) | Retrospective | Prostate | Sufentanil, NSAIDs, Ketamine, clonidine, EA | Increased risk with IV opioids |
| Lai et al. (2012) | Retrospective | Liver | GA<br>EA | Favors GA |

[a] EA favorable only in patient without metastasis
[b] EA favorable only in patient > 64 Y/O
[c] EA favorable only if started intraoperatively
[d] EA favorable only for rectal carcinoma
*EA* epidural analgesia, *GA* general anesthesia, *LA* local anesthesia, *PVA* paravertebral analgesia, *NSAIDs* non-steroidal anti-inflammatory drugs

because of the lack of consistency in the available results. Hopefully in the future, results of randomized controlled trial will shed more light regarding this matter.

### 9.4.3 Non Steroidal Anti-Inflammatory Drugs

Non-steroidal anti-inflammatory drugs (NSAIDs) may play a role in tumor progression and metastasis either directly via inhibition of cyclooxygenases (COX 1 and 2) and therefore prostaglandins synthesis, or indirectly through narcotic-sparing effects. Prostaglandins may affect immunity and inflammation by suppressing cell-mediated immunity both in vitro and in vivo (Chambrier et al. 1996; Elenkov et al. 2000; Faist et al. 1990). It is well known that PGs, especially $PGE_2$, have angiogenic properties. This effect can be blocked with NSAIDs. In rodent models NSAIDs have been shown to have both anti-tumor and anti-angiogenic properties. In an animal study examining rats inoculated with lung tumor cells, the authors demonstrated a 50% reduction in metastasis when the animals received the anti-inflammatory indomethacin. This reduction was further increased to 75 % with the addition of the β-blocker nadolol (Melamed et al. 2005). However, it appears that specific inhibition of the COX2 enzyme offers more benefit than non-specific inhibition of COX enzymes. The selective effects of COX2 inhibition was demonstrated by Farooqui et al. (2007). Moreover, the combination of β-blockers and COX 2 inhibitors was found in multiple animal models to improve immune competence and reduce the risk of metastasis (Benish et al. 2008; Glasner et al. 2011). In the clinical setting, the use of ketorolac was recognized to be associated with lower recurrence rates in patient undergoing breast surgery (Forget et al. 2010). However, this was not the case for patients undergoing prostate surgery (Forget et al. 2010).

In summary, the perioperative use of NSAIDs could potentially decrease tumor recurrence. Furthermore, the addition of a β-blocker to the NSAIDs regimen seems to confer more protection in animal models.

### 9.4.4 Other Modalities of Analgesia

Several modalities and regimens of analgesia could be used as an alternative to morphine and other opioids during the perioperative period. The majority of these modalities will serve to decrease the amount of morphine and opioids delivered at the time of surgery. These strategies include the use of $\alpha_2$ adrenergic receptor agonists such as clonidine and dexmedetomidine. The opioid-sparing effects of these drugs are well established. Clonidine is most commonly used to enhance the duration of regional anesthesia. Its intravenous use is associated with side effects such as hypotension and severe bradycardia. On the other hand dexmedetomidine offers the option of intraoperative use owing to its titrability, sedative effect and opioid-sparing effect. Nonetheless, $\alpha_2$ agonists seem to have tumor-promoting effects

(Bruzzone et al. 2008). Another attractive option is the use of neuropathic drugs such as gabapentin or pregabalin. These drugs belong to a family of anti-convulsant compounds largely used for chronic pain control, and have been advocated for use during the perioperative period to minimize intra-operative and postoperative opioids consumption (Bornemann-Cimenti et al. 2012). Finally, the perioperative use of β-blockers has been shown to reduce opioids consumption and, in animal studies, to limit tumor retention, as well as metastasis when given in combination with PG synthesis inhibitor (Melamed et al. 2005).

## 9.5 Conclusions

In addition to surgery, chemotherapy, radiation therapy, hormonal therapy, immunotherapy and other cancer treatment modalities, certain interventions during the perioperative period could also have a potential impact on long-term outcomes of cancer surgery patients, prolonging disease-free interval and overall survival of patients. Despite the accumulating evidence from cell culture experiments, animal experiment studies and retrospective clinical evaluations, we are unfortunately far from reaching recommendation regarding the anesthetic management of these patients. Whether interventions such a epidural analgesia, regional anesthesia and NSAIDs confer some degree of protection as compared to other types of pain management is still largely to be determined. This could be related to many factors such as tumor type, site, degree of invasion at the time of surgery. It is evident that randomized prospective trials (level I) are required before absolute recommendations are made.

## References

Afsharimani B, Cabot PJ, Parat MO (2011) Morphine use in cancer surgery. Front Pharmacol 2:46

Amato A, Pescatori M (2006) Perioperative blood transfusions for the recurrence of colorectal cancer. Cochrane Database Syst Rev 1:CD005033. doi:10.1007/BF02235262

Anderson SK (2005) Biology of natural killer cells: what is the relationship between natural killer cells and cancer? Will an increased number and/or function of natural killer cells result in lower cancer incidence? J Nutr 135(12):2910S

Azuma Y, Shinohara M et al (2000) Comparison of inhibitory effects of local anesthetics on immune functions of neutrophils. Int J Immunopharmacol 22(10):789–796

Bar-Yosef S, Melamed R, Page GG et al (2001) Attenuation of the tumor-promoting effect of surgery by spinal blockade in rats. Anesthesiology 94:1066–1073

Beilin B, Martin FC, Shavit Y et al (1989) Suppression of natural killer cell activity by high-dose narcotic anesthesia in rats. Brain Behav Immun 3:129–137

Beilin B, Shavit Y, Hart J et al (1996) Effects of anesthesia based on large versus small doses of fentanyl on natural killer cell cytotoxicity in the perioperative period. Anesth Analg 82:492–497

Ben-Eliyahu S (2003) The promotion of tumor metastasis by surgery and stress: immunological basis and implications for psychoneuroimmunology. Brain Behav Immun 17(Suppl 1):S27–S36

Ben-Eliyahu S, Shakhar G, Rosenne E et al (1999) Hypothermia in barbiturate-anesthetized rats suppresses natural killer cell activity and compromises resistance to tumor metastasis: a role for adrenergic mechanisms. Anesthesiology 91:732–740

Benish M, Bartal I, Goldfarb Y et al (2008) Perioperative use of beta-blockers and COX-2 inhibitors may improve immune competence and reduce the risk of tumor metastasis. Ann Surg Oncol 15:2042–2052

Biki B, Mascha E, Moriarty DC et al (2008) Anesthetic technique for radical prostatectomy surgery affects cancer recurrence: a retrospective analysis. Anesthesiology 109:180–187

Bone RC (1996) Immunologic dissonance: a continuing evolution in our understanding of the systemic inflammatory response syndrome (SIRS) and the multiple organ dysfunction syndrome (MODS). Ann Intern Med 125:680–687

Bornemann-Cimenti H, Lederer AJ, Wejbora M et al (2012) Preoperative pregabalin administration significantly reduces postoperative opioid consumption and mechanical hyperalgesia after transperitoneal nephrectomy. Br J Anaesth 108:845–849

Brittenden J, Heys SD, Ross J, Eremin O et al (1996) Natural killer cells and cancer. Cancer 77:1226–1243

Bruzzone A, Pinero CP, Castillo LF et al (2008) Alpha2-adrenoceptor action on cell proliferation and mammary tumour growth in mice. Br J Pharmacol 155:494–504

Cadet P, Mantione KJ, Stefano GB (2003) Molecular identification and functional expression of mu 3, a novel alternatively spliced variant of the human mu opiate receptor gene. J Immunol 170:5118–5123

Cassuto J, Sinclair R, Bondorevic M et al (2006) Anti-inflammatory properties of local anesthetics and their present and potential clinical implications. Acta Anaesthesiol Scand 50(3):265–282

Chambrier C, Chassard D, Bienvenu J et al (1996) Cytokine and hormonal changes after cholecystectomy: effect of ibuprofen pretreatment. Ann Surg 224:178–182

Christopherson R, Beattie C, Frank SM et al (1993) Perioperative morbidity in patients randomized to epidural or general anesthesia for lower extremity vascular surgery. Perioperative Ischemia Randomized Anesthesia Trial Study Group. Anesthesiology 79:422–434

Christopherson R, James KE, Tableman M et al (2008) Long-term survival after colon cancer surgery: a variation associated with choice of anesthesia. Anesth Analg 107:325–332

Coderre TJ, Katz J, Vaccarino AL, Melzack R et al (1993) Contribution of central neuroplasticity to pathological pain: review of clinical and experimental evidence. Pain 52:259–285

Delogu G, Moretti S, Antonucci A et al (2004) Apoptogenic effect of fentanyl on freshly isolated peripheral blood lymphocytes. J Trauma 57:75–81

Demicheli R, Miceli R, Moliterni A et al (2005) Breast cancer recurrence dynamics following adjuvant CMF is consistent with tumor dormancy and mastectomy-driven acceleration of the metastatic process. Ann Oncol 16:1449–1457

Dunn GP, Old LJ, Schreiber RD (2004) The immunobiology of cancer immunosurveillance and immunoediting. Immunity 21:137–148

Elenkov IJ, Wilder RL, Chrousos GP, Vizi ES et al (2000) The sympathetic nerve – an integrative interface between two supersystems: the brain and the immune system. Pharmacol Rev 52:595–638

Exadaktylos AK, Buggy DJ, Moriarty DC et al (2006) Can anesthetic technique for primary breast cancer surgery affect recurrence or metastasis? Anesthesiology 105:660–664

Faist E, Ertel W, Cohnert T et al (1990) Immunoprotective effects of cyclooxygenase inhibition in patients with major surgical trauma. J Trauma 30:8–17

Faist E, Schinkel C, Zimmer S et al (1996) Update on the mechanisms of immune suppression of injury and immune modulation. World J Surg 20:454–459

Farooqui M, Li Y, Rogers T et al (2007) COX-2 inhibitor celecoxib prevents chronic morphine-induced promotion of angiogenesis, tumour growth, metastasis and mortality, without compromising analgesia. Br J Cancer 97:1523–1531

Fleischmann E, Marschalek C, Schlemitz K et al (2009) Nitrous oxide may not increase the risk of cancer recurrence after colorectal surgery: a follow-up of a randomized controlled trial. BMC Anesthesiol 9:1

Forget P, De Kock M (2009) Could anaesthesia, analgesia and sympathetic modulation affect neoplasic recurrence after surgery? A systematic review centred over the modulation of natural killer cells activity. Ann Fr Anesth Reanim 28:751–768
Forget P, Vendenhende J, Berliere M et al (2010) Do intraoperative analgesics influence breast cancer recurrence after mastectomy? A retrospective analysis. Anesth Analg 110:1630–1635
Forget P, Tombal B, Scholtes JL et al (2011) Do intraoperative analgesics influence oncological outcomes after radical prostatectomy for prostate cancer? Eur J Anaesthesiol 28:830–835
Fuggetta MP, Di Francesco P, Falchetti R et al (2005) Effect of morphine on cell-mediated immune responses of human lymphocytes against allogeneic malignant cells. J Exp Clin Cancer Res 24:255–263
Glasner A, Avraham R, Rosenne E et al (2011) Improving survival rates in two models of spontaneous postoperative metastasis in mice by combined administration of a beta-adrenergic antagonist and a cyclooxygenase-2 inhibitor. J Immunol 184:2449–2457
Goldfarb Y, Ben-Eliyahu S (2006) Surgery as a risk factor for breast cancer recurrence and metastasis: mediating mechanisms and clinical prophylactic approaches. Breast Dis 26:99–114
Gottschalk A, Ford JG, Reglin CC et al (2010a) Association between epidural analgesia and cancer recurrence after colorectal cancer surgery. Anesthesiology 113:27–34
Gottschalk A, Sharma S, Ford JG et al (2010b) Review article: the role of the perioperative period in recurrence after cancer surgery. Anesth Analg 110:1636–1643
Gupta K, Kshirsagar S, Chang L et al (2002) Morphine stimulates angiogenesis by activating proangiogenic and survival-promoting signaling and promotes breast tumor growth. Cancer Res 62:4491–4498
Gupta A, Bjornsson A, Fredriksson M et al (2011) Reduction in mortality after epidural anaesthesia and analgesia in patients undergoing rectal but not colonic cancer surgery: a retrospective analysis of data from 655 patients in central Sweden. Br J Anaesth 107:164–170
Hanahan D, Weinberg RA (2000) The hallmarks of cancer. Cell 100:57–70
Hengartner MO (2000) The biochemistry of apoptosis. Nature 407:770–776
Hollmann MW, Gross A, Jelacin A, Durieux ME (2001) Local anesthetic effects on priming and activation of human neutrophils. Anesthesiology 95:113–122
Hong JY, Lim KT (2008) Effect of preemptive epidural analgesia on cytokine response and postoperative pain in laparoscopic radical hysterectomy for cervical cancer. Reg Anesth Pain Med 33:44–51
Iglesias M, Segura MF, Comella JX, Olmos G (2003) Mu-opioid receptor activation prevents apoptosis following serum withdrawal in differentiated SH-SY5Y cells and cortical neurons via phosphatidylinositol 3-kinase. Neuropharmacology 44:482–492
Ismail H, Ho KM, Narayan K, Kondalsamy-Chennakesavan S (2010) Effect of neuraxial anaesthesia on tumour progression in cervical cancer patients treated with brachytherapy: a retrospective cohort study. Br J Anaesth 105:145–149
Keh D, Boehnke T, Weber-Cartens S et al (2003) Immunologic and hemodynamic effects of "low-dose" hydrocortisone in septic shock: a double-blind, randomized, placebo-controlled, crossover study. Am J Respir Crit Care Med 167:512–520
Kehlet H (1989) The stress response to surgery: release mechanisms and the modifying effect of pain relief. Acta Chir Scand Suppl 550:22–28
Kelly G, Strasser A (2011) The essential role of evasion from cell death in cancer. Adv Cancer Res 111:39–96
Koodie L, Ramakrishnan S, Roy S (2010) Morphine suppresses tumor angiogenesis through a HIF-1alpha/p38MAPK pathway. Am J Pathol 177:984–997
Kundu JK, Surh YJ (2008) Inflammation: gearing the journey to cancer. Mutat Res 659:15–30
Kurosawa S, Kato M (2008) Anesthetics, immune cells, and immune responses. J Anesth 22:263–277
Lai R, Peng Z, Chen D et al (2012) The effects of anesthetic technique on cancer recurrence in percutaneous radiofrequency ablation of small hepatocellular carcinoma. Anesth-Analg 114:290–296

Landen CN, Lin YG, Amaiz Pena GN et al (2007) Neuroendocrine modulation of signal transducer and activator of transcription-3 in ovarian cancer. Cancer Res 67:10389–10396

Leo S, Nuydens R, Meert TF (2009) Opioid-induced proliferation of vascular endothelial cells. J Pain Res 2:59–66

Lewis JW, Shavit Y, Terman GW et al (1983) Apparent involvement of opioid peptides in stress-induced enhancement of tumor growth. Peptides 4:635–638

Lin X, Wang YJ, Li Q et al (2009) Chronic high-dose morphine treatment promotes SH-SY5Y cell apoptosis via c-Jun N-terminal kinase-mediated activation of mitochondria-dependent pathway. FEBS J 276:2022–2036

Lin L, Liu C, Tan H et al (2011) Anaesthetic technique may affect the prognosis for ovarian serous adenocarcinoma: a retrospective analysis. Br J Anaesth 108:814–822

Lutgendorf SK, Cole S, Costanzo E et al (2003) Stress-related mediators stimulate vascular endothelial growth factor secretion by two ovarian cancer cell lines. Clin Cancer Res 9:4514–4521

MacGregor RR, Thorner RE, Wright DM (1980) Lidocaine inhibits granulocyte adherence and prevents granulocyte delivery to inflammatory sites. Blood 56:203–209

Magnusdottir H, Kirno K, Ricksten SE, Elam M (1999) High thoracic epidural anesthesia does not inhibit sympathetic nerve activity in the lower extremities. Anesthesiology 91:1299–1304

Marx J (2008) Cancer biology. All in the stroma: cancer's Cosa Nostra. Science 320:38–41

Masur K, Niggemann B, Zanker KS, Entschladen F (2001) Norepinephrine-induced migration of SW 480 colon carcinoma cells is inhibited by beta-blockers. Cancer Res 61(7):2866–2869

McMillan DC, Wotherspoon HA, Fearon KC et al (1995) A prospective study of tumor recurrence and the acute-phase response after apparently curative colorectal cancer surgery. Am J Surg 170:319–322

Melamed R, Rosenne E, Shakhar K et al (2005) Marginating pulmonary-NK activity and resistance to experimental tumor metastasis: suppression by surgery and the prophylactic use of a beta-adrenergic antagonist and a prostaglandin synthesis inhibitor. Brain Behav Immun 19:114–126

Melchi CF, Mele A, Baliva G et al (1995) Prognostic value of anesthesia type for patients treated for cutaneous melanoma. Dermatol Surg 21:786–788

Mellon RD, Bayer BM (1998) Role of central opioid receptor subtypes in morphine-induced alterations in peripheral lymphocyte activity. Brain Res 789:56–67

Mikawa K, Akamarsu H, Nishina K et al (2003) Effects of ropivacaine on human neutrophil function: comparison with bupivacaine and lidocaine. Eur J Anaesthesiol 20:104–110

Moss J, Rosow CE (2008) Development of peripheral opioid antagonists' new insights into opioid effects. Mayo Clin Proc 83:1116–1130

Myles PS, Peyton P, Silbert B et al (2011) Perioperative epidural analgesia for major abdominal surgery for cancer and recurrence-free survival: randomised trial. BMJ 342:d1491

Oliveira GS, Ahmad S, Schink J et al (2011) Intraoperative neuraxial anesthesia but not postoperative neuraxial analgesia is associated with increased relapse-free survival in ovarian cancer patients after primary cytoreductive surgery. Reg Anesth Pain Med 36:271–277

Page GG (2005) Surgery-induced immunosuppression and postoperative pain management. AACN Clin Issues 16:302–309 (quiz 416–418)

Pasi A, Qu BX, Steiner R (1991) Angiogenesis: modulation with opioids. Gen Pharmacol 22:1077–1079

Pera M, Nelson H, Rajkumar SV et al (2003) Influence of postoperative acute-phase response on angiogenesis and tumor growth: open vs. laparoscopic-assisted surgery in mice. J Gastrointest Surg 7:783–790

Raven R (1990) The theory and practice of oncology: historical evolution and present principles. Parthenon Publishing Group, Park Ridge

Reiche EMV, Nunes SO, Morimoto HK (2004) Stress, depression, the immune system, and cancer. Lancet Oncol 5:617–625

Rosenberg SA, Lotze MT, Yang JC et al (1993) Prospective randomized trial of high-dose interleukin-2 alone or in conjunction with lymphokine-activated killer cells for the treatment of patients with advanced cancer. J Natl Cancer Inst 85:622–632

Sacerdote P (2008) Opioid-induced immunosuppression. Curr Opin Support Palliat Care 2:14–18

Sacerdote P, Manfredi B, Bianchi M et al (1994) Intermitent but not continuous inescapable foot-shock stress affects immune response and immunocyte beta-endorphin concentration in the rats. Brain Behav Immun 8:251–260

Sacerdote P, Bianchi M, Gaspani L et al (2000) The effects of tramadol and morphine on immune responses and pain after surgery in cancer patients. Anesth Analg 90:1411–1414

Salo M (1996) Cytokines and attenuation of response to surgery. Acta Anaesthesiol Scan 40(2):141–142

Schlagenhauff B, Ellwanger U, Breuninger H, et al (2000) Prognostic impact of the type of anesthesia used during the excision of primary cutaneous melanoma. Melanoma Res 10(2):165–169

Schmidt W, Schmidt H, Bauer H et al (1997) Influence of lidocaine on endotoxin-induced leukocyte-endothelial cell adhesion and macromolecular leakage in vivo. Anesthesiology 87(3):617–624

Seebacher C, Heubaum F, Kuster P et al (1990) Comparative analysis of narcosis and local anesthesia in surgery of malignant melanoma of skin. Hautarzt 41:137–141

Shavit Y, Martin FC, Yirmiya R et al (1987) Effects of single administration of morphine or footshock stress on natural killer cell cytotoxicity. Brain Behav Immun 1:318–328

Sinclair R, Eriksson AS, Gretzer C et al (1993) Inhibitory effects of amide local anaesthetics on stimulus-induced human leukocyte metabolic activation, LTB4 release and IL-1 secretion in vitro. Acta Anaesthesiol Scand 37:159–165

Snyder GL, Greenberg S (2010) Effect of anaesthetic technique and other perioperative factors on cancer recurrence. Br J Anaesth 105:106–115

Stein C, Rosow CE (2004) Analgesics: receptor ligands and opiate narcotics. In: Evers AS, Maze M (eds) Anesthetic pharmacology: physiologic principles and clinical practice. Churchill Livingstone, Philadelphia

Sueoka E, Sueoka N, Kai Y et al (1998) Anticancer activity of morphine and its synthetic derivative, KT-90, mediated through apoptosis and inhibition of NF-kappaB activation. Biochem Biophys Res Commun 252:566–570

Tegeder I, Grosch S, Schmidtko A et al (2003) G protein-independent G1 cell cycle block and apoptosis with morphine in adenocarcinoma cells: involvement of p53 phosphorylation. Cancer Res 63(8):1846–1852

Thaker PH, Han LY, Kamat AA et al (2006) Chronic stress promotes tumor growth and angiogenesis in a mouse model of ovarian carcinoma. Nat Med 12:939–944

Tsui BC, Rashiq S, Schoplfocher D et al (2010) Epidural anesthesia and cancer recurrence rates after radical prostatectomy. Can J Anaesth 57:107–112

Vallejo R, de Leon-Casasola O, Ramsun B (2004) Opioid therapy and immunosuppression: a review. Am J Ther 11:54–65

Wada H, Seki S, Takahashi T et al (2007) Combined spinal and general anesthesia attenuates liver metastasis by preserving TH1/TH2 cytokine balance. Anesthesiology 106:499–506

Welters I, Menzebach A, Goumon Y et al (2000) Morphine inhibits NF-kappaB nuclear binding in human neutrophils and monocytes by a nitric oxide-dependent mechanism. Anesthesiology 92:1677–1684

Wuethrich PY, Hsu Schmitz SF, Kessler TM et al (2011) Potential influence of the anesthetic technique used during open radical prostatectomy on prostate cancer-related outcome: a retrospective study. Anesthesiology 113:570–576

Yamashita JI, Kurusu Y, Fujino N et al (2000) Detection of circulating tumor cells in patients with non-small cell lung cancer undergoing lobectomy by video-assisted thoracic surgery: a potential hazard for intraoperative hematogenous tumor cell dissemination. J Thorac Cardiovasc Surg 119:899–905

Yanagi H, Sankawa H, Saito H, Likura Y (1996) Effect of lidocaine on histamine release and Ca2+ mobilization from mast cells and basophils. Acta Anaesthesiol Scand 40:1138–1144

Yang EV, Sood AK, Chen M et al (2006) Norepinephrine up-regulates the expression of vascular endothelial growth factor, matrix metalloproteinase (MMP)-2, and MMP-9 in nasopharyngeal carcinoma tumor cells. Cancer Res 66:10357–10364

Yardeni IZ, Beilin B, Mayburd E et al (2009) The effect of perioperative intravenous lidocaine on postoperative pain and immune function. Anesth Analg 109:1464–1469

Yeager MP, Colacchio TA, Yu CT et al (1995) Morphine inhibits spontaneous and cytokine-enhanced natural killer cell cytotoxicity in volunteers. Anesthesiology 83:500–508

Yeager MP, Procopio MA, DeLeo JA et al (2002) Intravenous fentanyl increases natural killer cell cytotoxicity and circulating CD16 (+) lymphocytes in humans. Anesth Analg 94:94–99

Yin D, Mufson RA, Wang R, Shi Y (1999) Fas-mediated cell death promoted by opioids. Nature 397:218

Yoshida AS, Tokuyama S, Iwamura T, Ueda H (2000) Opioid analgesic-induced apoptosis and caspase-independent cell death in human lung carcinoma A549 cells. Int J Mol Med 6:329–335

# Index



M.-O. Parat (ed.), *Morphine and Metastasis*, DOI 10.1007/978-94-007-5678-6,

## L



## M



## N



## O



## P

If you have any concerns about our products,
you can contact us on
**ProductSafety@springernature.com**

In case Publisher is established outside the EU,
the EU authorized representative is:
**Springer Nature Customer Service Center GmbH**
**Europaplatz 3, 69115 Heidelberg, Germany**

Printed by Libri Plureos GmbH
in Hamburg, Germany